# Medicine and the Christian mind

Edited by J. A. Vale

Second edition

D1440024

London

Christian Medical Fellowship Publications

© CHRISTIAN MEDICAL FELLOWSHIP, LONDON

*First Edition* 1975
*Second Edition* 1980


CHRISTIAN MEDICAL FELLOWSHIP PUBLICATIONS
157 Waterloo Road, London SE1 8XN


British Library Cataloguing in Publication Data
*Medicine and the Christian Mind*
1. Medical ethics    2. Medicine – Decision making
I. Vale, John Allister


ISBN 0 85111 971 9

*Printed by Stanley L. Hunt (Printers) Ltd.,*
*Midland Road,*
*Rushden, Northants*

# Contents

# Contributors

MONTAGU BARKER, MB, FRCP, FRCPsych, DPM

Consultant Psychiatrist, United Bristol Hospitals and Barrow Hospital; Clinical Lecturer in Mental Health, University of Bristol.

STANLEY BROWNE, CMG, OBE, MD, FRCP, FRCS, DTM

Director, Leprosy Study Centre, London; Consultant Adviser in Leprosy to the Department of Health and Social Security.

GEORGE CHALMERS, MB, MRCP

Consultant Geriatrician, Western Infirmary, Glasgow; Clinical Lecturer, University of Glasgow.

MURIEL CROUCH, MB, FRCS

Formerly Consultant Surgeon, Elizabeth Garrett Anderson Hospital, London and South London Hospital for Women and Children.

VINCENT EDMUNDS, MD, FRCP

Consultant Physician, Mount Vernon Hospital, Northwood, Middx.

The late IAN GORDON-SMITH, MB, FRCS

Formerly Senior Surgical Registrar, St. Mary's Hospital, London.

DOUGLAS JACKSON, MD, FRCS

Formerly Consultant Surgeon, Birmingham Accident Hospital and the MRC Burns Unit; Senior Clinical Tutor, University of Birmingham.

ALAN JOHNSON, MChir, FRCS

Professor of Surgery, University of Sheffield.

PHILIP KENNEDY, MB, MRCP

Consultant Neurologist, Southampton.

VICTOR PARSONS, DM, FRCP

Consultant Physician, King's College Hospital, London; Physician in charge, Renal Dialysis Unit, Dulwich Hospital, London.

GORDON SCORER, MBE, MD, FRCS

Formerly Consultant Surgeon, Hillingdon Hospital, Middx.

JOHN TRIPP, BSc, MD, MRCP

Consultant Paediatrician, Royal Devon and Exeter Hospital, Exeter.

CHRISTINE TUCK, MB, FRCS, MRCOG

Consultant Obstetrician and Gynaecologist, York.

ALLISTER VALE, MB, MRCP

Senior Medical Registrar, Guy's Hospital, London.

DUNCAN VERE, MD, FRCP

Professor of Therapeutics and Hon. Consultant, The London Hospital.

# Preface

The aim of the second edition of *Medicine and the Christian Mind* is the same as that of the first. It has been produced primarily to provide a short introduction to some of the problems faced by those embarking upon a career in medicine, though it should also prove of interest to members of the nursing profession.

Each of the contributors is well qualified by virtue of position and experience to write on the subjects covered. Between them they represent a wide field of medical and surgical practice. In addition, all the authors believe that the application of Christian principles offers the most reliable and convincing guidance in this sphere.

Several new chapters have been added and all other contributions have been revised. Sadly, Ian Gordon-Smith and his family were killed in a road accident in Thailand while Ian was working at Manorom Christian Hospital on secondment from St. Mary's Hospital, London. Ian is greatly missed.

It is a pleasure to acknowledge the help of several colleagues: Dr. Andrew Brown has designed the cover and general layout for both editions, and Mr. John Rivers has kindly seen the manuscript through the press. The Editor is most grateful also for the constant encouragement and advice of Dr. Douglas Johnson and Miss Muriel Crouch, FRCS, respectively the past and present Publications Secretaries of the Christian Medical Fellowship, but for whom this second edition might not have appeared.

London, 1980                          ALLISTER VALE.

# 1  The Christian role in medicine

Stanley Browne

THE title presupposes several questions. If there is a distinctive Christian role in Medicine, is there any point in maintaining it, or in trying to maintain it? Or, should this role be modified, or even, as some would suggest, abandoned, having outlived its purpose and its usefulness?

## The present situation

Modern medical practice in the West has its roots in mediaeval Christian belief. The early doctors of our era took over what was good in Greek medicine – the Hippocratic Oath, and the like – and added thereto the novel Christian motivation of care for the individual sick person. We have recently been reminded by such bodies as the World Medical Association, the World Health Organization and the United Nations that there is much in the morals and the ethics of ancient Greece and Rome to which we should do well to pay heed.

There are today many disturbing indications that certain principles of sound and ethical medical practice are being forgotten, wilfully neglected, and even repudiated. It is the convinced Christian who will in the last resort stand, and perhaps stand alone, for the upholding of these principles. It was the Christians, as Einstein reminded us some years ago, and not agnostic scientists or humanists, who dared to condemn (often at the cost of life itself) the excesses of Nazi materialism and racism. It was men of conviction and moral courage who stood up for principles that are today, once again, in danger of falling into disrepute or being repudiated by the vocal exponents of scientific humanism. Some of these principles may not be specifically Christian in their origin or application; but it is the present-day Christians who are being challenged in various ways to maintain these principles, which may otherwise go by default.

Is there, then, a distinctive role for the Christian who today finds himself in the world of Medicine, as student, practitioner or teacher? I submit that there is. What is at stake is deeper and greater than etiquette. It is more than the 'good life' and more than good medical practice. It is the profound ethics of our Lord's injunction – 'Treat others as you would like them to treat you.'[1] This includes every aspect of our relations with our patients – professional, social, cultural and spiritual. It includes investigation, research and treatment.

Although there is a distinctive role for the Christian doctor to fulfil in this age, we are nowhere called upon to conform to it in a stereotyped fashion. We are to use our training and gifts in the way in which God leads us. Far from being cast in the same mould, we each have some unique way of maintaining the distinctive task in Medicine.

## Christian character

The first and most obvious way is the maintenance of a distinctive Christian character. This will mean, in the first place, a conscientiousness in all that we do, in our whole practice of Medicine, a reliability in all aspects of our work, a thoroughness for instance in history-taking, in clinical examination and in the management of the patients entrusted to our care. This Christian character will show itself in the way we cope with the ordinary business of life, of getting on with others or joining in with them, not drifting with the stream but by being one with our fellows in all that is good. In our ordinary social contacts, too, I would deprecate strongly the mock piety of word, gesture and attitude that sets us apart in a holy huddle of like-minded friends. The spiritual influence of a Christian Union may sometimes be gauged from the degree to which its members participate in the sporting and other corporate activities of the Medical School. We must get to grips with the actual problems of our colleagues. This cannot be done if we keep ourselves apart. If our faith is a hothouse affair, and if we are fearful of the winds of change and the gales that may blow against it, then it is high time that we boldly face the fact and do something about it.

Christian character will manifest itself in our medical practice in a continuing willingness to go the extra mile for the sake of our patients. We shall take a real interest in the individual, by showing him genuine consideration and sympathy. We must regard him throughout not as a 'case' but as a person. The quality of our medical care is determined by our Christian principles. When we are meeting with patients (and with patients' relatives too, for we must not forget them) at perhaps a critical moment in their lives, that is, when they are facing the grim realities of life and death, what we *are* (as well as what we do and say) may count inestimably for their good or ill.

In our relations with colleagues, we are called to show spontaneously the Christian graces of true humility, sympathy and empathy. We must offer genuine friendship to the other man, finding out what he thinks and why. We need to be completely natural and outgoing.

Then, again, we must show a fearlessness in exemplifying and advocating the highest ethical standards in our duties, not 'toadying' to our chiefs or riding roughshod over those who work with us or under us. Similarly, in research, our inescapable duty is one of honest investigation, even if our work calls only for a critical reappraisal of accepted norms of diagnosis and treatment. The true Christian has openness of mind, honesty of purpose and reverence for what God allows him to investigate.

## Christian commitment

The second great contribution, I suggest, lies in Christian commitment. It will show itself in a response to the challenge to pioneer wherever there is a need in remote geographical areas, or in unattractive situations. We must accept, wholeheartedly, the Master's criteria of service and success – 'By losing his life for my sake, he will find it.'[2] When I recall the numerous mission hospitals that are now closing their doors for want of staff, and, at the same time, look back at the Christian medical students who at the time seemed so promising and who had promised their Master that they would devote their lives to His service, I am appalled and ashamed. If I had my own life over again, I can think of no more challenging and professionally satisfying task than to follow the Master's call to some specially needy medical sphere.

Such Christian commitment is displayed not only in medical work at home or abroad, but also in refusing to conform to the generally accepted standards, for instance the 'rules' of the 'rat-race'. I would not, of course, say a word against justifiable ambition, but the selfish and unscrupulous jockeying for promotion is quite foreign to the example and precept of our Master. There are far more important things in life than money or position. Let us by all means develop to the utmost the gifts with which God has entrusted us, but we must not confuse ambition with an unholy striving for a place in the sun.

I have mentioned money. It seems far removed from the ideals of service within a learned profession and a tradition of Christian culture, when doctors are seen by the public and the Health Department as being inordinately concerned about salary and conditions of service. The materialistic standards of today, the ordinary talk in the common rooms and medical clubs, the worship of goods and the standard of living – 'rich in things, and poor in soul' – all this seems foreign to the simplicity of the Master who left heaven in order to serve. Young Christians have a vital duty to help maintain the integrity of the Profession, and unselfishly to foster at all levels the Christian ideals of service.

## Christian applications

In the third place, our distinctive role is seen in the application of our Christian convictions to the burning questions of the day. We owe it to ourselves, to the public and to generations yet unborn to form with the greatest care our attitudes to topics that impinge upon medicine, ethics and religion. We must base our attitudes on facts rather than on will-of-the-wisp opinions, and build up for ourselves those standards of reference that will help us in grappling with new problems as they arise. In so doing, we shall prepare ourselves to meet the challenge of the humanist, the agnostic and the vociferous anti-Christian, as we meet them in the wards, in the common rooms and in medical practice at all levels.

It is becoming fashionable to ridicule and sneer at Christian beliefs. Those who uphold Christian standards are pilloried, or politely ignored. Rather than bow before the onslaught, we should take the war into the enemy's camp, graciously but with deliberation. Before we can battle effectively with any hope of success, however, we must ourselves be well prepared and well equipped, by reading, observation and discussion. In this way, we shall be able to help the undecided, the waverers and the decent uncommitted types among our fellow students.

Another way in which we can exteriorize this distinctive role is by keeping ourselves abreast of current thinking on major matters of ethical concern and by writing to the medical press, as occasion warrants, putting the 'other side', the side of the informed advocate of high Christian standards. We can in this way help our fellow medicals as they have to tackle the bristling moral and ethical problems raised in our modern society. I would urge that we do not cut ourselves off from them in the formative and deliberative years of our student days. There is need to strengthen the corporate advocacy of high ethical and Christian standards.

In the midst of the tumbling morals and permissiveness of today, we have a duty to become reasonably well informed about such matters as drugs and drink, sex and immorality, euthanasia, and abortion on demand. These are matters on which every doctor should have informed opinions, and on which he should be able to speak out. I fear that Christians are sometimes more concerned with orthodoxy of belief and its expression than with the matters that weigh heavy on the thoughts of our neighbours. Here lies the challenge of our time. We should meet it with a Christian commitment that will reinstate in the eyes of modern medical scientists a faith that is grounded in history and which can respond to the most penetrating demands of today.

**References**
[1] Luke 6:31.
[2] Matthew 10:39.

# 2 Should doctors play God?

Michael Webb-Peploe

I WONDER what your reaction is to this question. Do you become abstracted, philosophical, burdened by 'the weight of the awesome responsibilities given the doctor by modern technology', frightened by 'the incredible moral choices facing the Medical Profession today', to quote two phrases from a book with the title that is the subject of this chapter?[1]

'The incredible moral choices' and the 'awesome responsibilities' cannot be examined and dissected in a vacuum, because they always occur in the context of a human relationship between two people: a patient and his physician. We need therefore to seek to answer the following wider questions:

1. What is the role of the doctor?  Or, more personally: What are your aims and motives in Medicine?  Why do you want to be a doctor?  What sort of a doctor do you want to be?

2. What ought the doctor-patient relationship to be? Or, more personally: What is your attitude towards your patients?

With these wider questions in the forefront of our minds I want to examine three different applications of our title.

## A doctor's attitude to himself

A story is told of a consultant physician who lived some distance from the hospital where he worked. If in the morning he left home late to drive to the hospital he encountered a long traffic jam at a certain crossroads, and on such occasions it was his habit to overtake the queue of cars on the wrong side of the road, delicately dangling his stethoscope out of the car window. One morning, shortly after he had negotiated the traffic jam in this fashion, he was overtaken by a police car. As the police car went by its window was lowered and a blue-clad arm gently dangled a pair of handcuffs out of the window. History does not relate whether or not the physician took the hint; but the story illustrates very well that here was one doctor who thought that because he was a doctor he was above the rules and regulations governing lesser mortals. Such an attitude is one sure sign of a 'god-complex'. Avoiding such a complex involves being willing to subject ourselves to the ordinary disciplines of daily living: traffic discipline, the discipline of being on time for appointments, outpatients, ward rounds. It also involves the discipline of maintaining good working relationships with colleagues and nursing staff, of being accessible to patients and their relatives in times of crisis and emergency. We are not special, we are not exceptional just because we are doctors. Thomas Sydenham spelt this out very clearly in his 'advice to those entering the profession' when he wrote: 'The physician should bear in mind that he himself is not exempt from the common lot, but subject to the same laws of mortality and disease as others, and he will care for the sick with more diligence and tenderness if he remembers that he himself is their fellow sufferer.'

## A doctor's attitude to his patient

The sick come to us for advice on their medical problems; they do not come to us in order that we may make all their decisions, in order that we may run their lives for them. As a houseman, I remember looking after a young woman in her twenties suffering from angina due to familial hypercholesterolaemia. She was a nurse, and had planned to marry a missionary doctor and go with him to the Congo. Her physician, a very eminent cardiologist, told her that in no circumstances should she leave England, since the anticoagulant treatment she was receiving required very careful control. She broke off her engagement to the missionary doctor and stayed in England, and when I knew her, she was in great bitterness and agony of mind, wondering if she had missed God's will for her life. The true irony of this story emerges when one realizes firstly that anticoagulants are no longer considered an effective treatment for hypercholesterolaemia, and secondly, that a Congolese mission field diet would almost certainly have contained much less cholesterol than an ordinary English diet. As doctors, as mere men, we can never be omniscient, and to 'play God' in the lives of our patients is therefore to court disaster. It is our duty to give the best medical advice of which we are capable, to keep that advice up to date, and to help the patient to work out for himself the full implications of the advice that we have given him. The decision as to whether to accept or reject our advice must be left to the patient. To make the decision for him is an invasion of his personality. It diminishes him as an individual. Yes, by all means tell him what you think will happen if your advice is not followed, but be ready and willing to go on looking after him as best you can, even if he does not do as you advise.

There is no room for personal pride, for a 'god-complex' in the good doctor. Yet how often do we sacrifice our patients on the altar of our own self-esteem? Pride may be affronted when patients do not follow our advice. Pride may be offended when they ask for a second opinion. Pride may run away from situations that defy our medical skills: the incurably sick, the dying. In the face of inevitable defeat on a purely medical front, it is all too easy to leave it to the nursing staff and the relatives. But so often it is the incurable and the dying who most need our support and care. As Dr. Shirkey points out, 'The physician who seldom faces death may have fewer strengths than he who by trying experiences has faced it often. He must not steel himself with cold objectivity but, instead, with warmth and understanding. Distant objectiveness has no place when he leads his friends on their way, a journey which can be travelled emptily, or with dignity, pride, and for the greatest support of the dying. . . .'[2]

## A doctor's attitude to his colleagues

I get the impression that surgeons no longer throw instruments at junior medical and nursing staff with the same gay abandon as they did 25 to 50 years ago. Such tyrannical and unreasonable behaviour is likely these days to lead to a 'walk out' by the other members of the team. Medical practice is more and more a matter of teamwork, with no room for the temperamental and selfish *prima donna*. But, having said that, how do we treat our colleagues? (In this term I include medical and nursing staff, physiotherapists, medical social workers, dieticians, ward orderlies, porters – every member of the team caring for the patient.) If they are junior to us, do we regard them as subordinates, inferiors, inexperienced fools, or whipping boys when anything goes wrong? If senior, do we look on them as conservative stick-in-the-muds, ignorant old fuddy-duddies, and hopelessly behind the times? Or do we treat them, whether junior or senior, as valued members of the team, who have just as much, if not more, to contribute to the total care of the patient as we have? While some members of the team may appear to be more important than others, only rarely is any one member indispensable. Beware of the 'indispensability syndrome', of thinking that only you have the answer to the problem, that only you have the requisite skills to deal with a particular patient. The 'indispensability syndrome' is another sure symptom of the 'god-complex'.

## How do we avoid the God-complex?

I would suggest three words beginning with H – Humility, Humour, Humanity.

*Humility* – a constant awareness of our own ignorance, our own fallibility, and of how much we still have to learn. All the best physicians I have worked for were constantly asking questions, of junior staff, of technicians, of nurses, of anybody they thought might have the answers – and they were always prepared to say 'I don't know'. Humility shines through Sydenham's advice to those entering the profession: 'Whoever applies himself to Medicine should seriously weigh the following considerations: first, that he will one day have to render an account to the Supreme Judge of the lives of sick persons committed to his care. Next, whatever skill or knowledge he may, by divine favour, become possessed of, should be devoted above all things to the glory of God, and the welfare of the human race. Moreover, let him remember that it is not any base or despicable creature of which he has undertaken the care. For the only-begotten Son of God, by becoming man, recognized the value of the human race, and ennobled by His own dignity the nature He assumed.'

*Humour* – the ability to laugh above all at yourself. I am blessed in having a wife who, whenever she thinks I am taking myself too seriously, getting too big for my boots, gently but firmly pricks the bubble of my self esteem with the sharp pin of loving ridicule. This is a virtue to be highly prized in any doctor's wife!

*Humanity* – J. R. Batt (an American) in an Essay on Orwellian Medicine[3] writes: 'Unknown to most of us, there is evolving a new Medicine which seriously threatens our legally guaranteed democratic life style . . . Originally, our university medical centres were teaching hospitals where fledgling physicians learned to care for patients. These teaching hospitals were run by physician-professors who stressed the teaching of patient care techniques. However, over the last twenty years our nation's obsessive concern with scientific achievement has changed drastically the character of these institutions. The U.S. Government has made billions of dollars available for research in the basic life process sciences. Funds paid to medical centres for such research have increased 600% since the end of World War II. With the coming of this federal money, and funds from such private sources as the great drug manufacturing companies, corruption of the old style Medical School has become an accomplished fact. The research money and the power and prestige attached to the "big grant" made possible a distinct shift in the decision-making power within the medical centres. Increasingly the medical centres came under the control of the grantsmen. Consequently, today, the real way to a medical professorship, tenure, executive power, a handsome salary, etc., etc., is to do basic biological, chemical or physiological research – that is, be a grantsman. Patients and students are to be avoided like nuclear fall-out. This situation has, of course, turned our medical centres into tight little islands governed by men (minor gods) preoccupied with values which run contrary to the humane treatment of specific individuals suffering from illness.'

Before you dismiss this as a purely American phenomenon, let me point out that in Britain also devoted patient care is not the best 'road to the top'. Listen to what one disillusioned regional consultant has to say: 'We should have spent our time giving lectures, writing papers, and attending conferences. Our waiting lists would be miles long, we would get stacks of private practice, we would have made influential contacts, had the hospital rebuilt, and all got merit awards. Instead we made the mistake of treating the patients.'[4]

Some months ago a prominent Lebanese doctor came

to see me as a patient.  He had visited Britain often and was thoroughly familiar with the medical scene in this country.  At the end of our consultation he turned to me and said: 'What is happening to British Medicine and British Nursing?  It is losing all its humanity.'

*Should Doctors Play God?*  The answer is obviously 'No'.  But this is not the whole answer.  And now I want to turn the question round and ask reverently –

### 'How did God play doctor?'

In the Gospels, there is a wonderful story of a paralysed man and his encounter with Christ, the Great Physician.[5] Jesus is teaching the crowd, and debating with their religious leaders.  Suddenly there is an interruption. The roof of the house is being broken up, and a helpless paralysed man is lowered to the ground at Christ's feet. What were the Master's first words to this man who had so suddenly interrupted His teaching?  'Jesus seeing their faith' – that is, the faith of the sick man and of his four friends – said to the man, 'Take heart, my son.' The original Greek, literally translated, reads: 'Take courage child.'

Jesus, looking at this helpless man lying at His feet, saw that he was afraid, that there was something of the bewildered frightened child about him.  So His first words to the sick man were, 'Take courage child, don't be frightened, you are not alone, I am here, and I know your fear, your despair.'  Jesus sensed this man's agony of mind, and He hastened to relieve it.

But this was not all that He said, and His next words may come as a surprise to us.  They were: 'Your sins are forgiven.'  Jesus, looking at the broken man lying at His feet saw not only his fear, but also his guilt.  Face to face with the spotless Son of God that paralysed man realized as he had never realized it before that he was a guilty sinner in desperate need of forgiveness.  I know that these days it is not fashionable to talk about sin and guilt.  We prefer to use long psychological or sociological terms in an effort to persuade ourselves that really we are not responsible, it is not our fault, it is the fault of our parents, or of our education, or of the society in which we live. And yet, in our more honest moments of introspection, we have to admit that each of us has much of which to be ashamed, much to hide, much that needs forgiveness.

A perceptive doctor in charge of an intensive care unit has said that, in his experience, it is not so much the possibility of dying that distresses some of the patients in his care, but rather the thoughts of wrongs done and rights left undone, opportunities missed and human relationships tarnished and spoilt. I think that this is what St. Paul meant when he wrote to the Corinthians[6] that 'the sting of death is sin'. But, then, he went on – 'But thanks be to God who gives us the victory through our Lord Jesus Christ.'

Here was this paralysed man lying at Jesus' feet. You might well think that his most urgent need was for physical healing, for diseased nerves to regenerate and atrophied muscles to grow strong. But no, Christ looking at him saw that his first need was for peace of mind, and that his second need was for peace of heart – forgiveness of his sins. Only when He had dealt with these two aspects of the sick man's need did He finally say to him: 'Stand up, take your bed, and go home.' We are told that the helpless paralytic walked home rejoicing.

The frightened child had found a Comforter
The guilty sinner had found his Saviour
The helpless invalid had found the Great Physician.

Only if we have had this experience and have proved Him to be Comforter, Saviour, Physician, can we say with Paul: 'What a wonderful God we have. He is the Father of our Lord Jesus Christ, the source of every mercy, and the One Who comforts and strengthens us in our hardships and trials, so that when others need our sympathy and encouragement, we can pass on to them the same help and comfort that God has given us.'[7]

Human nature has changed little down the centuries. Many of our patients are just as frightened, just as oppressed by guilt, as was that paralytic. What have we to offer them? Is our Medicine going to become a 'power game' played against our colleagues, or the medical administrators, or the Government – a 'power game' in which the patient is a mere pawn, a population unit, a statistic to be manipulated in support of the doctor's bid for power, recognition, fame or money? Or is vital personal service rendered freely to suffering and needy human beings going to be the hallmark of the Medicine we practise? The only motive force powerful enough to achieve this sort of service is obedience to Christ's new commandment – 'that you love one another even as I have loved you'.

### References

[1] Frazier C. A. *Should doctors play God?* Nashville, Tennessee: Broadman Press, 1971.
[2] Shirkey H. C. Facing the inevitable. In *Should doctors play God?* Nashville, Tennessee, Broadman Press, 1971.
[3] Batt J. R. Hippocrates as 'Big brother'. In *Should doctors play God?* Nashville, Tennessee. Broadman Press, 1971.
[4] Anon. Forgotten exiles in Castleport. *Br. Med. J.* 1974, 1: 569-570.
[5] Matthew 9:1-8; Mark 2:1-12; Luke 5:18-26.
[6] 1 Corinthians 15:56,57.
[7] 2 Corinthians 1:3,4. Living Bible.

# 3  Doctor in the making

Douglas Jackson

DOCTORS are made, not born; this gives hope to those of us who feel we have still some way to go. A good doctor is a combination of scientist, healer, friend, social worker and technician. It is difficult to combine so many attributes; it is surprising how many do so successfully.

The making of a doctor, I suggest, is based on three foundation stones or accepted values; and, in the building that is raised on these, one should be able to distinguish at least two types of architecture or life-styles. Let us first look at the three personal values.

## Respect for truth

*Learn it*

All their lives doctors have to gather facts – signs, symptoms and investigations; they have to weigh these facts, act on them and assess the results. So it is essential that we fill our minds with knowledge early in our training. A student's first duty is to study; incidentally, you will never learn as easily again. Postgraduate study follows, not the minimum for examinations, but the maximum for our patients. The mind is not a box that we can overfill, as a student suggested to me recently; it is a computer, and we can only get out of it what we have properly fed into it.

## Discern it

'Discrimination' is a discredited word today because of its association with race or sex: but has not discrimination always been a sign of maturity? Learn not to accept all that is spoken confidently with authority, whether it be a political manifesto or a medical advertisement. There are different types of truth – historical, experienced and spiritual, to mention only three. Historical truth must be accepted on trust from historians and may save us from repeating the mistakes of the past. Personal experience may be true, genuine and very convincing, but it may be completely misinterpreted. It may be helpful or, on the contrary, damaging to character and good living. Spiritual truth deals with such questions as 'Why am I here?' 'Is there a God?' 'Can I know Him?' and 'Am I responsible to Him?' Only God can answer some of these questions and He has done so in the Bible. Are we trying to discern the truth, or are we ignoring great aspects of it, imagining they are worthless or will cease to exist if we do not consider them?

## Face it

Truth, in the abstract, may be a fascinating intellectual exercise; but it is not emotive or dynamic. For that, we must apply it to ourselves and those around us. Doctors have to handle the truth with their patients. Often it it unpalatable truth – strong and dangerous stuff, which can plunge them into acute anxiety or depression. I hope we shall all help our patients face it and handle it wisely and bravely; but, if we are going to do so, we ourselves must learn to face truth with intellectual honesty and not avoid it. The worst pretence is to deceive ourselves.

27

## Respect for people and personality

*People, not things*

All their lives doctors have to work with people – old and young, rich and poor, bright and subnormal, friendly and aggressive. Have you noticed how easy it is, when we are busy or preoccupied, to stop thinking of patients as people, and to think of them instead as cases, diagnoses, clinical problems or disordered mechanisms? But it is a person who is asking for our help and putting his life in our hands. As Paul Tournier, a well-known Swiss psychiatrist, has emphasized, 'Our patients want us to know all about their diseases, but they also want to be understood as persons.' It is true that in anatomy you have to start by studying the body as a thing: in physiology you study the interaction of mechanisms; in pathology you study living and postmortem disease; in sociology you study the behaviour patterns of elements in society. All these we need to know; but, when we practise Medicine, we are face to face with a person – often a frightened person in great trouble, a person who is in the dark and looking for someone he can trust. We work with people, not 'clinical material'.

*Unique, not uniform*

Not only should we respect people as persons, we should respect their personality. Every person is an individual. Just as every snow-flake has a unique crystalline pattern under the microscope, and every leaf of every tree has a different shape and marking, so God has made people with infinite variety. Each one is unique, each is 'one off'. The Apostle Paul repeatedly likened the ideal Christian society to the human body; this is a medical illustration which should appeal to us.[1] Each individual is a single part – an eye or ear, a hand or foot. Each is dependent on the others; none should have a superiority complex, saying, 'I don't need you'; none should have an inferiority complex and opt out, saying, 'I'm only a clumsy, flat foot. There's nothing I can do.' The pattern and plan is one of 'variety in unity for full activity.' This unity is certainly not uniformity.

The same principle applies to Christians as to society at large. When a man becomes a Christian, his mind and basic personal make-up do not change. If he had a second-class brain, he does not become a genius; if he was an introvert, he does not become an extrovert. A hundred Christians are not supposed to look like a page of postage stamps; we are not supposed to model ourselves on each other. Why, then, do we have this individuality? Not so that we can 'do our own thing'; this is man's trouble – we have already 'turned everyone to our own way'. Our individuality is to enable us to serve Jesus and help others in an absolutely unique way due to our God-given individual insights, understanding and gifts. We can each play an individual, but complementary, part in God's eternal purposes for the world. We each need to develop an individual dependence on the Lord Jesus, and then learn how to work synergistically with others. We see this often in the body: for the flexor muscles of the fingers to work strongly and effectively, the dorsiflexors of the wrist must work too. Both need to be under the control of the brain. Reflex activity, without going through the brain, is not a very high order of life!

## Respect for excellence

*Patient or self?*

If lives are going to depend on us, surely we must try to be as able and effective as we can be in our work. In these days, some are apt to question whether there is any need to do more than 'get by'. 'Surely competition implies succeeding at someone else's expense,' they tend to say; and 'Isn't personal ambition the cause of many evils?' Well, of course, ambition can sometimes be a great vice, and if it is self-centred it certainly will be. A doctor who has a selfish ambition to make a lot of money and wield influence and power will be a menace to his patients and colleagues; he will be tempted to trample over others for his own profit. With this attitude in mind, the prophet Jeremiah wrote, 'You seek great things for yourself. Leave off seeking them.'[2] But ambition can also be a virtue: it is perhaps because many of us have no high and holy ambition to be used by God in this world and generation that He is unable to use us in places of influence and responsibility. Behind all disciplined skill and training there must be a wish to excel; the alternative is mediocrity. Our safeguard with ambition in Medicine is that it should be patient-centred, not doctor-centred. 'How can I give my patients a better service?' rather than, 'How can I get more out of it?'

## God or man?

Intellectual honesty and the avoidance of pretence have already been mentioned: moral integrity is as important and as difficult to maintain. It is so easy to find an excuse to do what is pleasant or profitable, even when we doubt the propriety of that particular course of action. Two questions have been suggested as tests which we can apply personally when faced with difficult choices. First, when ambition beckons along some profitable path we can usefully ask ourselves, 'In whose eyes am I seeking to be successful; in God's eyes or man's?' Jesus had outspoken criticism for those who loved the praise of men more than the praise of God. The second question, valuable perhaps as we seek God's guidance about what to do with our lives and medical training is, 'For whose benefit am I qualifying (or practising)?' God has a plan for each of our lives and, in the final assessment, no other course can compare with it. He has His own individual ways of showing each of us His plan and what our priorities should be; but He expects us to ask for His guidance and to obey when He leads.

There are also two distinct aspects of living: discipline of myself and involvement with others.

## A disciplined, balanced life

The first life-style which needs to be learned in the making of a doctor is one of self-discipline. Because it is a life-long lesson each of us needs to start at it right away. It has four ingredients – none of them incompatible with laughter.

*Work*

I apologise for mentioning work again! Work is absolutely indispensable for a happy, fulfilled life as any severely disabled or unemployed man will tell you. Doctors are tremendously privileged to have such varied and satisfying work. Unless you are one of those who tend to become over-anxious about their work, learn to work hard because it increases your capacity. Rightly approached, examinations can be quite a helpful stimulus to work. Learn to use the various stresses of life to develop your character and ability. Soon you will find that some of the particular strains will cease to be felt as pressures because you will have grown and matured to accept them as normal. But, most important, *having worked – play*!

*Play*

Play at something; something you like and not too seriously. We all know of people who work and worry until they crack up. Everyone has a weak spot if the stress becomes great enough. It may be anxiety, depression, an ulcer, migraine or just becoming irritable and bad-tempered. Some use drugs or alcohol to escape. The safety valve is play or relaxation. Open-air exercise is one of the best forms, but you may prefer music, skating, photography, natural history or . . . whatever. Christians especially need mind-broadening interests. The word 'Puritan' today is often used to describe a narrow-minded, bigoted type of Christian, such as the later Puritans seem to have become; but the early Puritans were large-minded people, widely educated in music, the arts and literature. A Christian, if he has the opportunity, should be open to all that is good and excellent in the truest culture of body and mind.

*Home*

Few doctors escape the conflict between responsibility for their patients and for their families. Inevitably these claims conflict at times, and we must try to give each its due priority. Since this, too, is a life-long problem, we should start to face it in student days. Some who read this may be away from home for the first time. Keep in touch with a short note or 'phone call, and a visit when you can. It will bring real joy and encouragement at home, more than you think perhaps. If you get something out of it yourself, that is a bonus!

*Worship*

For a Christian there is an inner life with the Lord Jesus behind all his other activities. This also needs time each day if we are going to keep spiritually fresh and alive. Life has been likened to a three-legged stool where the legs represent body, mind and spirit (our relationship to God). Some people care for their minds but not their bodies, and are physically unfit; others are entirely devoted to personal fitness and sport, all muscle and little intellectual activity. It is just as easy and common to go through life with the third leg missing which makes us unbalanced and spiritually dead; or to have it an inch too long, and that's a caricature of a Christian! To be a whole, mature person we need to have all three aspects of our lives developed, and this includes a real personal relationship with the Master, speaking to Him in prayer and hearing Him speak from the Bible each day. Most Christians find it necessary to make this their highest priority. When we live like this there is little distinction between religious and secular living. Our daily work is as much an act of worship as verbal praise if offered to our Lord thankfully, and, in this way, we can thank Him 'not only with our lips, but in our lives . . .'. Medical life, of course, is busy and full of urgent calls, but it is important that we do not let the urgent crowd out the important.

## Getting involved

If this disciplined, balanced attitude relates to our inner life-style, 'getting involved' should characterize our outer life-style in society. In its simplest form this means learning to make warm human relationships. Some people, by nature and upbringing or due to some unfortunate experience, find it hard to make friends. Others are afraid that, if they give themselves to other people, things will get out of hand and become too costly in time and effort. Whatever the cause, if we feel weak in this respect we should try to improve, because it will become later a big part of good medical practice. If you are in your first year and still feel lonely, offer someone *your* friendship. Find someone you think you can trust, who will take you as you are, and will not use or manipulate you – someone in the hospital Christian Union perhaps – and ask them round one evening to coffee. My own advice is to avoid exclusive one-to-one relationships early on if you want to get the most out of university life, but this is just a personal view. The important thing is to get mixing.

Also, of course, a Christian will want to get involved in some form of Christian work and witness in the hospital during the week and in a church at the weekends. At certain periods in life, such as before exams, we may feel that we must shut down and concentrate on medical work wholly. University life, however, is a splendid opportunity to learn with other Christians how to study the Bible and apply it to personal life, ethics and politics; even more, we can learn how to share the life-changing message of Jesus and His love with other people. Christians need each other's friendship: a single piece of coal burning in a grate will soon go out, but two or more will go on burning brightly together for hours.

Once qualified, whether you like it or not, your patients will be looking to you to guide them in their personal problems and calamities – as human beings, not mindless machines. We all need help at times, but we also need to learn how to give it in an *acceptable* way.

## In conclusion

In matters of attitude and behaviour it is always interesting for a Christian to consider how our Lord would have thought and acted in the circumstances. You will remember that, after washing His disciples' feet, He told them, 'I have given you an example, that you also should do as I have done to you.'[3] Note then how these attitudes and life-styles that we have been considering are illustrated by Christ's own example.

In His temptations in the wilderness,[4] Jesus held fast to the truths of the Old Testament in spite of fierce temptations to be independent; and, later, in conversation with the woman at the well,[5] He felt it necessary to lay His finger gently but firmly on an unpalatable truth in her life. John described Jesus as 'full of grace and truth'.[6]

Then there was the incident when the scribes and Pharisees brought to Jesus the woman who had been caught in adultery.[7] With masterly dignity He put the forgiveness and reformation of this despised woman before exaction of the extreme penalty for breaking the law. He put the person before the principle, though He upheld the principle as well in His last words to the woman.

Jesus had no selfish ambition, but we can see His God-centred ambition as He affirms, 'My food is to do

34

the will of Him who sent me, and to accomplish His work.'[8]  Jesus nourished His own relationship with His Father, going up into the hills by Himself to pray after a heavy day.[9]  With unobtrusive discipline He balanced the claims of work,[10] rest,[11] family[12] and worship[13] in His own life, while all the time He was never too busy to get involved with others.[14]

It is not surprising, I suppose, that the Great Physician shows the makings of a doctor *par excellence*.

### References

[1] 1 Corinthians 12:12-27.
[2] Jeremiah 45:5.
[3] John 13:15.
[4] Matthew 4:1-11.
[5] John 4:16.
[6] John 1:14.
[7] John 8:1-11.
[8] John 4:34, 6:38; Luke 22:42.
[9] Matthew 14:23.
[10] John 9:4.
[11] Mark 6:31.
[12] John 19:26-27.
[13] Luke 4:16.
[14] Matthew 9:36.

### Further Reading

Short D. S. *Medicine as a vocation*. London: CMF Publications, 1978.

# 4 Clinical training

Victor Parsons

THE purpose of this chapter is to expose some of the hazards and opportunities of clinical training. In recent years the transition from preclinical to clinical and preregistration training has become smoother and the abrupt change from the purely university disciplines of preclinical studies to the more applied techniques of clinical medicine has tended to disappear. The intention is to engage in a continuing appreciation of the study of man from all aspects, biochemical, mental or spiritual, from the first year through to qualification, specialization, and beyond.

This will come about by the constant application of the earlier scientific disciplines to the contemporary problems of modern medicine, with their ethical problems raised at an early stage and their limitations clearly appreciated. Many students entering a period of clinical studies find their vivid exposure to disease and death as disturbing as the attitudes of their more senior colleagues to the vocation of Medicine are enervating. For some it takes time to adapt to what, in effect in other disciplines, is a period of postgraduate training. The increased freedom for study, the minimum of compulsion and the complexity of the problems of individual patients make it an almost uncharted sea. It is my purpose to erect 'marker buoys' to the main channels.

## Vocation: sentiment or signpost?

One such is a fresh assessment of the purpose of and vocation to Medicine. The 'erosion of vocation' is a common phrase difficult to measure, but felt as a genuine tendency by many clinical teachers. The increase in cynicism that has been measured[1] may stem from the fact that the few real successes of general medicine have to be set against the rising percentage of incurable, geriatric and chronic psychiatric patients in the general wards. Another factor is the increasing tendency for patients to be managed by a team and for decisions to be made 'in committee' so that the students' opinion weighs lightly, even if it is invited. This lessens the sense of responsibility for the management of the patient and of personal involvement in his care. The student is unable to help the patient's anxiety with any degree of authority. He may find himself unable to join in the general attitude to the patient with incurable or terminal illness. Although he may find satisfaction in the fullest documentation of the patient's history and the opportunity of kindness to the patients allocated him, the rewards are meagre. This situation is often reversed when the student becomes resident, when opportunities increase and, at last, he feels his vocation again.

Part of this erosion can be resisted by the Christian in his willingness to see how his beliefs influence his attitudes and actions in the face of illness and death. He must work out afresh his vocation and where he feels he can contribute most. Decisions are made around this time about the type of practice he should take up after qualification. Many Christians enter medicine with the conviction that this profession will give great opportunities for the redemption of the individual, or their ideal goal may be that of becoming a medical missionary. As

37

training goes on, opportunities for widening the Christian's contribution to medicine occur. The student may be attracted, more to improving the total situation, whether in correcting the 'diseases of choice' such as obesity, or preventing heavy smoking and alcoholic habits (which invite the inevitable epithet of a 'do gooder'), or in following the challenges of some specific research which may lead to the alleviation and prevention of particular diseases. In these latter situations the importance of Christian belief, with its eternal perspective and its elucidation of the meaning of illness and death, must be worked through by the individual.[2]

## Mastery

Another goal is mastery[3] of the skill of Medicine. This mastery gives satisfaction and the form of enjoyment which only comes from tasks well done in any profession or trade. It provides momentum to immerse oneself in the business of the various clerkships within hospital and in the appointments in general practice and community health. Mastery comes not only from the enthusiastic gaining of knowledge, but from repeated history-taking, examination and investigation until it becomes like knowing and using fluently a new language. The synthesis of the unique mass of data into a whole picture for each patient is a never ending task of infinite variety. To the patient himself it is never routine, and if the doctor plays his part in interpreting the disease to him, opportunities for personal contact are not lost as they might be if the patient were regarded as just 'another case'. The possibility of redemption of the individual in the face of terminal illness presents the Christian with the challenge of answering the question, 'To what purpose is this waste?' Nor need the mastery stop here, for behind every illness are the more creative possibilities of research and prevention which may be an increasing preoccupation of medicine in the future. From these can emerge reconstruction and a new understanding, if the clinician is not content with just diagnosis and treatment.

Mastery is linked to professional expertise. The present tendency to quantify professional activity, to delineate hours of work, to institute 'call back pay', all suggest that the profession is one of limited commitment. Rather one should look on the profession as giving fulfilment through the practice of well learned skills, and the rewards those of a task well done, rather than the means to an assured income, with 'industrial action' as an option to be exercised.

### Apprenticeship

Some think that this word should be quietly buried with the past, like 'barber surgeons'. However, many of the ways of dealing with patients are learnt by seeing other doctors in action. Often unconsciously the student finds himself absorbing their attitudes and values. This can be seen by the extraordinary influence James Bovell had on the young William Osler,[4] who described him as 'one in whom there was all one could desire in a teacher – a clear head and a loving heart'. From him Osler gained an intense interest in natural history and philosophy, and he was able to say of James Bovell and William Johnson that to them 'I owe my success in life – getting what you want and being satisfied with it.' From contact and friendship with such teachers in the apprenticeship system of the wards and clinics and beyond, much more is learnt than just the techniques of contemporary medicine. Among my own teachers I cannot forget two whose unconscious influence is still powerful; their approach to the history of disease, their immense care in the choice of words in telling the patient about his illness and the incredible ability to go on and on in keeping the highest standards right to the end of the longest day were unsurpassed. Ideally there should be opportunity for an interplay of ideas between teacher and student. This comes from the development of joint research projects at an early stage, from small tutorial classes and from the membership of clubs and societies which have meetings on a variety of subjects beyond the field of medicine.

One of the features of the present discontent among younger members of the Profession is the lack of guidance in the choice of postgraduate study and the failure of senior members in the profession to appreciate their needs and problems. These are signs of the breakdown in the apprenticeship system and may be related to the increasing numbers of students and the increased load of committee work which senior members are asked to undertake. Nevertheless the answer often lies in the student's approach. Some draw back from the exposure which is involved in true apprenticeship.

## Communication

This subject seldom appears in a medical school's curriculum and yet it plays an increasing part in the development of the 'good doctor'. The latter can be defined as one who 'knows his stuff' (knowledge and skills) and can 'relate well'. This ability to relate well, to communicate, will be the special concern of the Christian who will be used to manipulating concepts such as 'caring for', 'fellowship' and 'relationships'. At the lowest level this may represent just good manners and, at the highest, the care and love that goes into any relationship. Perhaps no feature marks out the good doctor more than the ability to communicate to those around him, whether it be colleagues, nurses or patients. A Christian should have the advantage in his training of coming alongside people, sitting where they sit, seeing needs above his own, and in his willingness 'to go out of his way' in his concern. It involves more than just getting on well with people as there will be a desire to be truthful in each situation and not just to opt for a 'quiet life'.

Communication is difficult to teach as such. How

'to speak the truth in love' is the ideal; but many will opt for some form of a compromise as easier. Particularly difficult is the case of the dying patient. Much has been written on this subject which will be helpful to the student.[5] The secret lies in spending more rather than less time with such patients, and showing an interest in what they are feeling at this very difficult and possibly lonely time.[6]

## A social sense

Doctors for the most part are individualists, who carve out a niche in society where they hope to be secure. At the same time they wish to be needed and to feel faintly indispensable. Often the student gains the impression that diagnosis and treatment are all that is required from the adequate physician or surgeon. It must be conceded that in the final examinations not much more is required. The diagnosis, however, must not only include 'How?', but the more difficult question 'Why?' For the patient and his family, the latter is often more important. Medical educators hope that in the future more attention will be paid to the social causes behind many of the diseases which keep our wards so busy today. Examples such as bronchitis, atheroma and peptic ulcer reveal how little we really know about the causes and the fundamental prevention of these and other diseases which stalk society today. The clinical years are not too early to start to wonder not only how they can be cured, but also how they can be anticipated and prevented.

The clinician's strong sense that he enters too late on the scene must drive him back to investigation and the possibility of action, which will be far removed from 'just picking up the bits'. An appreciation of the doctor's part in the prevention and anticipation of disease is best seen in the field of nutrition and the increasing interest in social psychiatry. It is often difficult to remember that the study of the environment and 'people in the mass' may sometimes be a more appropriate study than of the individual patient. This is specially so for those who feel that if only the individual is put right, the rest will look after itself. Yet (without detracting from true concern and involvement with the individual) some balance must be struck between the pressing needs of the various communities which make up our society. It seldom occurs to the student (unless he has lived in a tropical country) that his training may fit him just as well for seeking to change the environment as picking up the casualties in a faulty one. In the developing countries and perhaps in our own in the future, the emphasis will shift from the cure of disease to the promotion of health.

Although this concept may seem a long way off from the curriculum of today's student in training, it needs to be introduced as early as possible if more workers are to enter what some regard as, and some even hope will remain, the 'Cinderellas' of the profession. By all means let the molecular scientific end of the spectrum have its full play. Its rewards are apparent for all to see. Yet the interaction of people, working conditions and the fabric of society are equally fit fields for study, especially by those whose concern is to serve mankind as fully as they are able.

## Self, peer and teacher assessment

The knowledge of how one is progressing in the general flow of information gathering is an important, continual feature of education at any level. Numerous chances are now given to the student to assess his progress by self-administered questionnaires, multiple choice question examinations and the writing up of case histories. Much of this can be done at the student's own speed, but there are advantages in getting one's peers to scrutinize and criticize one's progress.[7] One way in which this can be done is by the use of the clinico-pathological conference (CPC) which originated when a law student lived with a medical student in Boston and the medical student heard the law students setting each other trial situations. The CPC remains a regular feature of the *New England Journal of Medicine* and of other journals.

## Making the most of the time

Tensions between competing disciplines and habits are a natural consequence of the freedom given to the student in these years, which contrasts with the more rigid preclinical courses which kept within the timetable of the academic year. From these tensions intellectual and moral growth is possible.

Right at the centre is the problem of organizing work and leisure, practical work and book work with the demands of competing communities, to all of which the student may belong simultaneously. It is a characteristic of living in a large town that an individual may belong to three community networks – those where he works, sleeps, and spends his weekends. He may belong to a student body where he lodges, a hospital firm or team, and to his home, which may perhaps be the most tenuous link. He may need to identify himself more closely with one than the other and the choice may be a painful one. Much will depend on whether he still lives at home, where opportunities are usually found at weekends in helping in the local church fellowship. During the week the Christian Union will need and give help. Living in lodgings, or in a Hall of Residence, he will have to attach himself to the local church or hospital chapel. There is much to commend the latter as it will provide support and opportunities for prayer on behalf of those he sees and talks with every day.[8]

No matter how good the clinical staff, the large range of patients available and the splendid library facilities, the student must be an active gatherer of knowledge. Very little absorption takes place without 'active transport'. Another factor that sometimes takes students a long time to appreciate amid all the discussions concerning vocation, ambition and guidance is that what matters is *work today*, not next year, when they qualify or settle down. The quality of daily work is the key to making the most of these years. A little personal research and introspection (with or without a stop watch) may be revealing and lead to a change in habits which are imperceptibly inherited from those around and before us.

Surveys over a whole week have shown that at least two-thirds of the day are spent in sleeping, eating, domestic duties, travelling and leisure, leaving *at most* eight hours for work in hospital and school. Of these eight hours some are already occupied by compulsory courses, lectures and demonstrations leaving some room for personal initiative. Clerking on the wards, attendances at emergency and outpatient departments can take up to twenty-four hours in a well planned six-day week, leaving eighteen hours a week for rounds, lectures, tutorials and talking shop with teachers and fellow students. What is left goes in reading and in research into particular problems. These figures are a very rough guide of what some students actually do. The variation between individuals is often a factor of two or three. They take into account, however, periods of hospital residence, when the daily average of time spent in hospital at work, may reach much higher values. There is a tendency for an increasing amount of leisure time to be available as the week goes on, leaving Sunday free for activities of any kind.

A sane balance must be achieved between practical skills and sheer gathering of information which involves reading and library work; but few students realize early enough that over 75 per cent of their examinations are designed to test information recall. Without this basic material, the foundations on which to build clinical expertise are going to be at least shaky, if not anecdotal. The constant referral back from clinical experience to reading is essential even in the first year of clinical work, when the books used earlier have often thankfully been put away. To have read about a patient's condition before the ward round is as valuable to the student as it is unnerving to the teacher.

One illustrative check on the time factor, and a possible stimulus for work, is to keep a diary. This need not necessarily be the daily sort, although this can be filled in for a week or two to get the feel of one's working capacity. It can also record questions which are unanswered, ideas to be worked out and, on occasion, ethical situations for which there seems no 'set' answer. Later these may be added to projects for research and solution. Over a year or two this kind of record can throw up enough material to sustain and increase one's momentum. Above all else, considerations of the use of time will continue to be a problem for the rest of one's life. The satisfaction of working out some plan at this stage will give confidence later when situations and circumstances may change quickly.

## The use of leisure

Leisure time is to be guarded and planned but perhaps in not such detail. Travelling in large cities is a serious leisure waster, as are poorly run committee meetings and unrestricted television viewing. Recreation comes into leisure time. No-one should grudge eight hours a week, but again the individual demand varies and many seem content with a moderate degree of physical fitness. Sunday has its special claims on the Christian in worship and helping in various activities. Leisure has a more positive aspect *still*, what Pieper[9] has called 'a time for wonder and marvelling' in contrast to attitudes of total work. These are times for drawing back from activity to gauge the whole picture from a distance; to ask questions which have neither simple nor static answers and may not be easily expressed to another person. Questions such as – 'What am I?' 'Where am I going?' 'What am I trying to do in this particular community?' Perspective of this sort may be gained by particular leisure activities, varying from music to bird watching. Why such activities bring with them a sense of proportion and gladness is difficult to define, but this lies at the basis of true leisure. It corrects the tendency to cynicism, which can occur so quickly in all of us.

## Vacations and elective periods

Perhaps no professionals need their vacations more than doctors. This is related to their being 'on call' and having the problems and needs of patients continually before them. When the legitimate chance comes 'to get away from it all', it is taken with both hands. This opportunity to live a different life usually involves travelling and meeting a new community. Students now have more openings than ever before through the various exchange schemes, Voluntary Service Overseas and elective periods mostly away from hospital and the usual curriculum. Apart from these special times, the shorter vacations give further chances to maintain friendships outside the world of medicine which keep things in perspective.

**References**

[1] Eron L. D. In, *The effects of medical education on attitudes in the ecology of the medical student*. Ed. Gee G. H. and Glaser F. J. Evanston, Illinois: A.A.M.C., 1958.

[2] Elphinstone A. *Freedom, suffering and love*. London: SCM Press, 1976.

[3] Coade T. F. *The burning bow*. London: Allen and Unwin, 1966.

[4] Cushing H. *The life of William Osler*. London: Oxford University Press, 1925.

[5] Twycross R. G. *The dying patient*. London: CMF Publications, 1975. Soell D. *Suffering*. London: Darton, Longman and Todd, 1975. Craig M. *Blessings*. London: Hodder and Stoughton, 1979. Gover G. *Death, grief and mourning*. London: Cresset Press, 1965.

[6] Saunders C. In, *Religion and Medicine*. Vol. I. Ed. Melinsky M. A. H. London: SCM Press, 1970. Lay P., Spelman M. S. *Communicating with the patient*. London: Staples Press, 1967. Bird B. *Talking with patients*. 2nd edition. Philadelphia: J. B. Lippincott, 1973. Lucas K. A. *Giving and taking help*. Chapel Hill, University of North Carolina Press, 1973. Mac-

Namara M. Talking with patients: some problems met by medical students. *Br. J. Med. Ed*, 1974; 8:17-23.

[7] Helfer R. E. Peer Evaluation, its potential usefulness in medical education. *Br. J. Med. Ed*, 1972; 6:224-231.

[8] Autton N. *Pastoral care in hospital.* London: SPCK, 1968.

[9] Pieper J. *Leisure the basis of culture.* London: Faber and Faber, 1952.

# 5  A basis for medical ethics

Muriel Crouch

MANY of those who have been impressed by the high standard of patient care exercised by the majority of doctors, the sanctity of the doctor-patient relationship, and the safeguards for the individual which are written into the practice of research, are often not aware of their source. They have regarded such terms as 'the sanctity of life', 'the preservation of life', 'the alleviation of suffering' and 'the rights of the individual' as inherent in medical ethics and have not stopped to consider from whence they have been derived.

Historically, at least in the West, the progress of Medicine has been closely bound up with the practice of the Christian Faith. This has taught that the dual purpose of Christ's ministry was to preach and to heal. His compassion and care for the most helpless and diseased, the deformed and the handicapped, and the infinite value He placed on the individual are reflected in His command to His apostles to 'heal the sick, cleanse the lepers, raise the dead and cast out devils'.[1] Such injunctions as that of James 1:27 make care of the orphan and handicapped a special responsibility of the followers of Christ, and a number of the greatest advances of medicine and surgery have sprung from a truly

Christian compassion.[2] Douglas Jackson comments: 'In this country at present, as far as can be told, our stated medical ethics are in full accord with orthodox Christian beliefs.'[3] But what some of us have failed to realize is that we are living on borrowed capital. Glanville Williams writes: 'This feeling, among those who do not subscribe to any religious faith, may sometimes be a legacy of their Christian heritage. . . . It may also originate in part from that inherent awareness of God's will which the Bible teaches is present in all men.'[4]

## The current crisis

The nature of ethics has been defined as the 'guiding principles and motive forces behind action'. We are faced today not so much with the question of whether there is an ethical basis for medical practice as with a choice of several approaches which demand our urgent and earnest consideration. Our generation has seen 'the climate of opinion going away repeatedly, and in different ways, from the previously accepted Christian standards'.[3] Rapid scientific and technological advance has put unparalleled powers in the hands of men, just at a time when the previously accepted moral and spiritual laws are being discarded. Seldom in the last two centuries have the traditional Christian view of man, the sanctity of human life and the value of the individual been so universally questioned.

While Science and its discoveries are neutral, the uses to which they may be put vary widely and, indeed, may be entirely opposed to each other. Thus, in the medical sphere, our newly found powers may be used for the preservation of life or for its destruction, for the increase of its quality or for the prolongation of its misery. It is no good imagining that as practising doctors we have no need to concern ourselves with the crucial problems of ethics. Many have anticipated a conflict which is surely coming, if for example, religion is to be regarded as a 'disease, a dangerous neurosis'. The humanist states 'Christian beliefs no longer carry conviction for the nation as a whole. Many thoughtful and responsible parents and teachers are in grave doubt about the truth of these doctrines. . . . It is now widely accepted that there is a common pool of human moral principle which need not in anyway be based on religious beliefs.'[5] It might be interesting to trace how much of this 'pool' ultimately stems from the Christian faith!

Although in many branches of Medicine, as for instance in research, Christian belief forms the basis of an ethical code, yet in others we are already feeling the impact of divergent beliefs, so that Christians begin to find themselves at variance with some of the current medical opinion and practice. For example, in the matter of abortion, the change in the climate of opinion is generating new problems for convinced Christians, who have high standards in relation to the indications for termination of pregnancy. Hence, we must be aware of the magnitude of the issues at stake, and of the degree of importance which we must attribute to our basic beliefs. As Douglas Jackson has said 'If the standard is to be safe in the future, we should be sure of the foundation truths on which it is based – that they are God given and permanent. It is the compelling sense that we must submit to the Author of those beliefs, when it is neither fashionable nor profitable to do so, that is the real safeguard of the patient, for it is this which gives the will and the power to live up to the standard.'[3]

## The need for convinced beliefs

As doctors we deal with people, with life at its conception and birth, with its quality, its preservation, its prolongation and its end. For the unbeliever, life has but two dimensions, physical and mental, and it is terminated by physical death. For the Christian, life has another dimension which supersedes the others in importance and quality, and which is not ended by death. Further, in dealing with problems of ethics we need to know what are basic Bible principles and what are customs derived from those principles. It is necessary to distinguish between what are moral laws, permanent and binding on all men, and what are social regulators adapted for a particular time, society or circumstance.

Clear thinking, too, is essential because we all suffer from the tendency to argue from the particular to the general and to be swayed by our immediate sympathies rather than by our basic convictions. Even for the mature Christian there are areas of overlap, where two opposing principles must be held in tension, and where the right course of action lies somewhere between the two. Such is the problem which faces us when the due relief of suffering might lead to the shortening of life.

Moreover, we are all in danger of oversimplification of rules. We long for clear-cut detailed instructions to which we can adhere – without the effort of thinking, or the responsibility of deciding. Such was the pitfall confronting the humanist who, asked by his TV interviewer what he would teach his children, replied 'Never do anything which hurts someone else.' A fair enough instruction if we know what constitutes the 'hurt'! Yet who more often than the doctor has to be cruel to be kind, and to inflict suffering in order to cure? Similarly, who more often than the Christian knows that the road to man's highest fulfilment – a restored fellowship with God – is often thorny and found only through suffering and the facing of unpalatable facts?

## The Christian ethic

We need to review and redefine the Bible's principles which have formed the Christian's basis for medical ethics in the past, and to measure against them some of the current beliefs which have given rise to the changing climate of opinion.

### Our view of God

As Christians we believe in God as Creator.[6] The dis-

51

coveries of Science far from undermining our belief, confirm it and enhance the glory of His wisdom and power. Furthermore, we know that He is not merely an 'Influence' but a Divine Person who has chosen to reveal Himself through His created universe,[7] through history and through the Person of His Son.[8] He has even revealed to us the purpose of His Creation, for 'The whole universe has been created through Him and for Him'[9] and 'By Thy will they (i.e. all things) were created and have their being.'[10] He holds the ultimate issue of life, death and eternity and He will finally vindicate His honour.[11]

God has shown to us that His purpose for man is a personal relationship with Himself 'Whom to know is life eternal.'[12] Only as man is brought into such a relationship by God's redemptive intervention, will he be fulfilled, find happiness and his true destiny and share in the purpose of God. To this end God has given us a Moral Law which is 'an expression of what God demands of man; it derives from God's own character, permanent, unchangeable, and eternal as God Himself – applicable to all men'.[13]

In marked contrast is the humanist view. To him there is no Creator God; 'man is the resultant of evolutionary processes – but having evolved he is now powerful in relation to his environment and responsible for his own destiny. Master of his world, he is responsible for his future'.[5] Man, then, in the humanist's view, holds the issues of life and death. He believes that he will increasingly do so. With the powerful weapons of transplant surgery, genetic change, and the biochemical creation of life he claims to be near the secret of immortality. Moreover since there is no God, there is no Divine source of truth. 'We accept nothing as revealed truth.' So there is no knowledge beyond what can be discovered by the reasoning powers of man. Again, 'we do not believe there is any ultimate purpose in life nor think there is any point in looking for one'.[5] What a tragedy if man should be able to shape his evolution and destiny and yet have no purpose for which to use them! He has the power to go somewhere, but has nowhere to go!

Finally in this connection, the humanist believes in no external authority, and no moral law, but only 'the laws and institutions devised by society to prevent chaos'. Small wonder that we are living in a society where laws are being changed to suit the convenience of the majority! Even smaller wonder that we are beginning to experience and witness the chaos that the laws are devised to prevent!

## The divine will and purpose

These differing views of God and His relation to His created world have a profound effect on our attitude to our research and medical practice. The Christian must be humble in His approach to a God-centred universe, he admits the limitation of his finite mind and the perversion of his motives. He wants to find God's purpose for human life and will seek a mandate for its control. The humanist regards the universe as man-centred, for man to use as is convenient. Baroness Wootton has epitomised the position as 'We no longer ask what is pleasing to God, but what is good for man.' As Victor Parsons comments – 'She overlooks the possibility that what is pleasing to God is good for man.'[3]

The Christian, on the one hand, looks to God as his only hope, asks for His help, and seeks to keep the moral law. He thus fulfils his responsibility towards God in his control of life, while the humanist, on the other, looks to man alone, is devoid of any Moral Law and lacks a sense of responsibility to any but himself. Thus 'As a rule of thumb to live by we believe those actions which lead to unhappiness are bad. This "open society" aims at promoting in a commonsense way, freedom and happiness for as many as possible without favouring a particular group.'[5] Alas, that the humanist has underrated the selfish nature of man and overlooked the fact that 'the fault, dear Brutus, is not in our stars, but in ourselves that we are underlings'. The prospect of life as it is, rendered immortal by man, is too horrifying for contemplation. The Christian can thank God that He has ordained it otherwise,[14] and can rejoice that his ultimate future depends not on scientific advance, but on the fact that his name is written in the Lamb's Book of Life.[15]

## The nature of human life

The Christian doctor needs, too, to be clear in his mind regarding the nature of man's life. Many would define 'life' purely in biological terms believing that human life does not differ in essence from animal life. But the Christian believes that man is unique, because he has been made in 'the image of God'.[16] This uniqueness is evidenced by his self-consciousness, his discernment of moral values and ability to make moral judgments and, above all, to know God and to have a personal relationship with Him of dependence, trust and obedience.[13] This essential self-consciousness gives rise to the view that 'Life is something which is experienced.' Similarly, Duncan Vere defines life as 'personality', either at present or as a future potential, and 'we may recognize personality (i.e. ability to respond to God) by the ability, however slight, to respond to us'.[3]

This concept of 'potential' is important, hence life defined in this sense, though lacking now, as in the fetus, may be gained later, or, as in the unconscious patient, regained later. The Moral Law as revealed in the Bible reflects the value of human life in the eyes of God. God has always held man responsible for the life of his fellow man.[17] Premeditated murder demanded the death sentence. The sixth Commandment, 'Thou shalt not kill,' was underlined by Jesus, Who had come not to destroy the law but to fulfil it. He regarded the motive behind murder to be as culpable as the deed itself.[18]

54

The Christian knows that this life is only part of a much greater whole, and that death is only an incident, though an important one, in a larger life. Beyond it lies the judgment[19] and, for those who know Him, a wonderful future in God's presence.[20] On the other hand, the humanist does not expect to 'survive death in any sense at all' (Ayer). Such a divergence of belief cannot help being reflected in a divergence of medical practice.

## Motivation and power

The Christian Faith provides us with ethical principles on which to base our medical practice. It also holds before us a standard of integrity and selfless service which should characterize the handling of our patients. It also produces the loyalty and sincerity which should mark our relationships with our colleagues. But, in addition, it offers us the enlightenment and guidance of the Holy Spirit in the problems which inevitably face us. We are called to undertake a daily walk with a living Lord Who imparts to us the power to put into practice the convictions that we hold. He offers a relationship with Himself for which there is neither parallel nor substitute.

**References**

[1] Matthew 10:8.
[2] Capper W. M. *Some great Christian doctors*. London: CMF Publications, 1959.
[3] Edmunds V., Scorer C. G. *Ethical responsibility in medicine*. London: Livingstone, 1967. (The respective chapters are under the names of the contributors to whom reference is made.)
[4] Romans 2:15.
[5] The parts in inverted commas in quotations attributed to Humanists have been taken from booklets and leaflets issued by the British Humanist Association.
[6] Genesis 1; Colossians 1:16; John 1:3.
[7] Romans 1:20.
[8] Hebrews 1:1-3.
[9] Colossians 1:16.
[10] Revelation 4:11.
[11] Ephesians 3:9-11.
[12] John 17:3.
[13] Jackson D. *The sanctity of life*. London: CMF Publications, 1962.

[14] Genesis 3:22-24; 1 Corinthians 15:21-24.
[15] Revelation 21:27.
[16] Genesis 1:26,27; Genesis 2:7.
[17] Genesis 4:10, 9:5.
[18] Matthew 5:17,21,22.
[19] Hebrews 9:27.
[20] 1 John 3:2; Revelation 21:1-7.

**Further Reading**

Crouch M. *Imparting ethics to medical students.* London: CMF Publications, 1977.

Jackson D. M. *Professional ethics – who makes the rules?* London: CMF Publications, 1972.

Scorer G., Wing A. Eds. *Decision making in medicine – the practice of its ethics.* London: Edward Arnold, 1979.

Bliss P. B., Johnson A. G. *Aims and motives in clinical medicine – a practical approach to medical ethics.* London: Pitman Medical, 1975.

# 6 Talking with patients

Gordon Scorer

WHEN patient and doctor meet there is an interchange
of words. One is in personal need; the other has the
means to help. If the need is trivial the encounter is
short and words are then few, and few is enough. On
the other hand, the meeting may be the beginning of
long friendship set in a professional context in which
conversations are long and deep. Words are the cement
and strength of each encounter. Be they grave or gay
the meaning is always important, because illness is
always important.

## A helpful attitude

If reports from patients are true it seems that the doctor
sometimes fails in his efforts to convey information, or
consolation, or even interest. Thoughtless words can so
easily be damaging – 'words as hard as cannon balls'.
Considered words, precisely tailored to anticipate the
anxious fear, can help and heal. Paul advised Christians
about how they should talk with people. The same
advice is well suited to the doctor's consulting room:
'Let your speech always be gracious, seasoned with salt,
so that you may know how you ought to answer everyone.'[1]

What is gracious speech? Surely it is that the speaker is using words not merely from a sense of duty but out of respect for, and interest in, the listener. Gracious words warm the heart as well as inform the mind; they are acceptable and appreciated.

Such speech should not stand alone; it needs to be 'seasoned with salt'. Salt has two purposes. It brings out the flavour of the food and, in the long term, it acts as a preservative. Perhaps, in medical practice, our conversation needs to be spiced (not overloaded) with humour and homeliness, so that our patient can the more easily grasp our meaning. Important too is the need for our counsel to be incorruptible and such as will make it easier for the patient to want the right things in life.

It is, of course, in the Christian context – and presumably in the defence of his faith – that Paul ends his advice with the comment '. . . that you may know how you ought to answer everyone' – or better, as in the NEB, 'Study how best to talk with each person you meet.' Conversation in the consulting room needs to be natural and relaxed, but we can afford to sit back from time to time and see if we are making our interviews as effective and helpful as they ought to be. It is a salutary experience when a patient comes back and repeats to us what we told him a year ago or ten years ago. It is surprising sometimes to learn of the impression we gave or of the nonsense we apparently talked.

## Economy of words

A physician speaks with authority. He must do so, for he has had many years of training to give him the basic knowledge of how the body works in health and in disease. The patient is not only in need, but is more or less ignorant of what is going on within him. He comes to the doctor because the doctor is an expert and he expects an authoritative answer. This means in the first place we need to be sure of our facts before we make a pronouncement, and, secondly, we need to be careful in the choice of words we use. A doctor's word is final in the clinical context unless the patient chooses to question it and seek a second opinion. If we are not certain of diagnosis and treatment we need to say so. If time alone will solve a problem we need to say so. If a second opinion is needed it is better to swallow our pride (if we are allowing it room in our hearts) and mention the need for further help before the patient does.

The imparting of gratuitous medical information is better avoided. It is wiser to wait till the patient gives a lead and asks. Many are satisfied with simple two-syllable explanations in two sentences; a few want to know more. It is not that we majestically preserve our professional secrets, but rather that we speak to the intelligence of the patient and give him what he needs in order to make his own way forward to full recovery. A learned judge, in a celebrated case of operative damage to the recurrent laryngeal nerve, said he did *not* think it necessary to warn a patient of all the possible complications of an operation. He regarded a doctor who did this as going beyond his duty.

## Tips from clinical experience

Here are a few points about talking to patients. Most of them are glimpses of the obvious, but they can so easily be overlooked:

*Look the patient in the eye*

Not a studied gaze to embarrass, of course, but at least a reassuring welcome as he comes nervously to sit down opposite you. A frequent glance as you speak and then a momentary strong look when you stand to say goodbye. At least the patient then leaves you knowing he has met a human being and not a robot behind a counter. Incidentally, you can learn so much about a patient from his eyes, quite apart from the clinical information they give. Character is more quickly revealed here than elsewhere. Mouth and hands and gait also speak volumes – but that is another story.

## Get alongside the patient when you talk

It is an old trick of the interviewer to put his patient in a strong light and himself stand or sit where the light is behind him and his face cannot so easily be seen. This is gamesmanship and not always right in clinical medicine. In talking to a patient it is often prudent to get down to the same level as he is, to sit by a bedside or to go down on your haunches in talking to a child. It puts them at their ease. Better still move around occasionally.

## Speak slowly

It is surprising how often we speak too fast for patients – particularly the old – to understand. Simple sentences in simple words and repeated in the same interview are often needed. There is no need to shout – that is rightly considered rude – but it is surprising how many old people are a little deaf and politeness forbids some of them from asking you to repeat yourself. Clear and simple speech needs to be cultivated and it is a great asset to be able to describe complicated procedures in one-syllable Anglo-Saxon.

## Be human

Perhaps the lightest and simplest touch of humanity is to pick up something of interest in a patient's story and digress for a moment. A holiday? – Where did you go? The family? – How many have you? How are they doing? Your work? – Tell me a little about it, I'm interested.

This reveals medical competence as well as humanity, for a patient is far more likely to expose his own problems if he knows his physician is a ready and gracious listener. What a sad indictment it is when we hear someone say 'I can't talk to my doctor '

## Curb impatience

Temper your busy-ness and learn to listen. If a patient is anxious, she needs to be allowed to talk, she needs to be drawn out and encouraged to express her fears. If a patient is angry he needs to get it off his chest – let him talk: you will win a friend. If a patient is a chatterbox, beware – she may be wasting your time. Some patients need to be interrupted politely but firmly – 'but, wait a minute, let's get to the point. What is it that is *really* troubling you?' – or – 'Look, if we get that pain of yours cured will you then be perfectly fit?'

On the whole we need to listen more than we do, and at least to offer opportunity for them to talk. 'Was there anything else that you wanted to mention?'

## Beware of clichés

As doctors most of us are far too prone to lapse into them. They are the mark of slip-shod thinking. Here are some common ones: 'Don't worry.' (Probably the patient had never thought of worrying until you mentioned the word.) 'Take it easy.' (What *does* that mean?) 'You'll be all right.' (Does that mean 'We hope you will survive this drastic treatment' or 'We know you will make a complete recovery'? There is a world of difference.) 'Don't eat too much.' (Feeding habits need to be precisely investigated before such advice is of any value.)

'When men talk too much, sin is never far away: common sense holds its tongue.'[2] Too many words and too much exhortation confuse. A few well chosen words addressed to the main point at issue go much further than much half-baked medical jargon buttered over with clichés.

## Always keep a step ahead

Anticipate your patient's next probable anxiety and his likely course ahead. It is a wonderful comfort to a patient if he is told what to expect during his course of treatment. A neurologist examined a patient after he had become paralysed as a result of a haemorrhage into the spinal cord. After careful assessment the neurologist outlined a programme showing how recovery of function would occur, how long it would take and what would be the likely residual disability. The patient was then well armed to face his prolonged convalescence with courage and confidence. It is a wise doctor who thinks ahead for his patients.

### Keep to the truth

Lies, especially white ones, breed like mice. On the other hand, it is not right for the doctor to be driven by an over sensitive conscience and destroy a patient's hope by saying too much. If it is a matter of a bad prognosis or a probable fatal outcome, it is always better to wait until the patient gives a lead. And in any case it is always right to let the patient know that however difficult or ineffective the treatment may be, *you* will always be available to help and to do something. Incidentally, of course, if you say you will do something for the patient, don't forget to do it and do not break your word. Almost always in terminal illness the best treatment we can give our patient is a regular dose of our interested selves.

### Christian witness

Should the Christian speak of his Lord and Saviour? Yes, certainly, as occasion offers. It is better to be brief unless the patient specifically asks for a discussion. A word of personal testimony does not offend. A single challenging verse or thought about Christ in the context of the patient's need is more valuable than a theological debate. Firm friendship with the hospital chaplain or a local Christian minister means you can work together for those in need. He can often do much more than you, after you have given the introduction. But it needs to be said again and again, that the doctor's task is first and last, and all along, to be a good doctor – *not* an evangelist.

## Beware of arrogance

Pomposity and hypocrisy are the errors of a cultured élite. It is all too easy to adopt the pose of infallibility and inwardly preen ourselves when success and popularity come our way. Others detect the dread signs in us before we notice them ourselves, for our speech betrays us. It is a betrayal of our calling as Christians and as doctors. It is an attitude of mind that needs to be avoided at all costs. After all, what have we, as doctors or as Christians, that we have not received from others. To them be the honour.

**References**

[1] Colossians 4:6.
[2] Proverbs 10:19.

# 7  Suffering and death
Muriel Crouch

IN considering a subject of this sort, there inevitably
spring to our minds pictures of patients we have seen,
some mishandled, others well handled; some wanting to
know the truth, others not wanting to know; some taking
it well, others badly; some for whom death was quick
and merciful, and others for whom it was prolonged and
agonizing.   We find ourselves confused by the variety in
temperament of our patients and the multiplicity of the
problems and situations facing us, and we are often
undecided as to the course of action we should take in
face of the varying needs before us.

It is, however, important that we avoid the pitfall of
considering particular cases, before establishing general
principles; and rather than discussing right action we
should at first establish right attitudes – our own right
attitudes – in the whole matter of suffering and death.
The establishing of right thinking is important for two
particular reasons: firstly, if we are people of sympathy
and imagination (and it is to be hoped that we are) we
lie between the Scylla of being steadily broken by the
suffering of others, and the Charybdis of protecting ourselves by a hard impenetrable crust which makes us
callous regarding the needs of others.   In either case we

are rendered useless. Right thinking however, will help us as Christians to find adequate resources from outside ourselves, so that while giving out all the time, we are nevertheless not depleted nor worn out, but rather act as channels for the grace and power of God. 'Over-powering strains balanced by limitless resources; when these two work together as God means that they should, they make giants in power and millionaires in grace and experience.'

A second danger is that of retaining a student view-point too long. The student is essentially an observer, and stands in the gallery of the theatre, watching the operation and the drama played out. Many retain their student attitude long after qualification, and watch their patients struggling, suffering, living and dying, never realising that their problems are ours, their suffering may be ours, and their death sooner or later will be ours, perhaps sooner rather than later. Inciden-tally it is worth noting that with the upsurge of television programmes portraying hospital life, many of our patients have joined us in 'the gallery' and, with their detached view of life, have become infected with our disease!

## The basic problem

In considering this subject we must turn to the basic problem confronting us. How can the facts of suffering and death be compatible with the belief that God is a God of love? This is not merely of academic impor-tance, for only recently has the author heard of a medical student who has jettisoned his faith, having foundered on this very rock that 'there cannot be a God of love when there is human suffering as I see it in the wards'. This question poses several others. These we shall consider in turn.

## Suffering in the world – whose fault?

If God cares why did He do what He did? Why did He

put suffering into the world? Or did He? Was it His primary purpose? If not, how can we say He is omnipotent? From the Genesis record it would seem that God's creation was perfect, 'It was excellent in every way.'[1] And man He made 'like His Maker' a reasoning moral being, with mastery over the rest of creation, abundant provision for all his needs and a capacity for fellowship with his Maker.[2] But by Genesis 3, we find a very different world in which the seeds of all the ills of modern society are apparent. Already man is ashamed of himself and afraid of his Maker,[3] not only blaming others for his foolishness, but the God who gave them, 'it was the woman you gave me' he said.[4] The first mention of 'intense pain and suffering'[5] is as a direct result of the woman's disobedience towards God, while man's relentless struggle to survive, his sweat and toil to extract a living from the soil, his frustration with 'thorns and thistles', and finally his losing battle with disease and death, all result from his yielding to the temptation of the woman to disobey God's laws.[6] In the subsequent chapters we find the beginnings of a deceit, jealousy, pride, hatred and murder with which we are all too familiar.

From the record it is apparent that suffering and death were the result of man's action taken independently of God, as he deliberately forsook his role of obedience to and co-operation with God. How did such action come about? Why did man do it? Why did he then, and why has he ever since, set his heart on things that satisfy only his animal appetites, appeal to his aesthetic senses and give him a sterile knowledge and power without the moral stature to use them aright? 'When the woman saw that the tree was good for food and that it was a delight to the eyes and that the tree was to be desired to make one wise she took of the fruit and ate and she gave some to her husband and he ate.'[7] It is enigmatic that man so often loves best the things that destroy him or spoil his life, the over indulgence in food, the excess of alcohol, the wrong use of sex, the abuse of drugs, and the craving for smoking. He is prepared to give everything he has in pursuit of pleasures that are transitory. A hint at the answer is found in 1 John 2:16 'All these worldly things, these evil desires – the craze for sex, the ambition to buy everything that appeals to you, and the pride that comes from wealth and importance – these are not from God.' Where then are they from? 'They are from this evil world itself.'

## The origin of evil

But what made it evil? Whence temptation? Granted that man disobeyed and brought about the whole train of events which has afflicted the human race ever since, what made him do it? At the beginning of Genesis 3, we find that man acted as he did because he was tempted to disobey God by an evil being. Someone outside himself appealed to his natural desires and through them undermined his loyalty to God. The methods of approach of that being are well known to all of us in experience. Firstly, he tempted man to doubt God's Word, 'Really?' he asked 'God says you mustn't eat any of it?';[8] next, to deny its truth, 'That's a lie! You'll not die!'[8] and, finally, to doubt God's love and wisdom towards us. He implied that God's laws are intended to limit and curtail our happiness rather than to promote it. 'God knows very well that the instant you eat it you will become like Him, for your eyes will be opened – you will be able to distinguish good and evil.'[8]

The Bible says little about the way such a being came into God's created world. Perhaps this is not surprising since it is primarily a record of God's dealing with man and not of His handling of the universe. Nevertheless most of us have no difficulty in believing that there is such a spiritual being opposed to God. We are aware of the reality of temptation in our lives and the constant downdrag from even our human ideals. Moreover, as we look at the world we see cruelty and inhumanity which can be described as diabolical. Men seem to be swept along by a power outside themselves. Indeed, in our generation we are aware of those who are deliberately setting out to communicate with the powers of evil and even giving their heart's allegiance to such. The existence of such a being may be the answer to the problem that troubles many. It may explain the disruption of the whole created universe indicating that man's moral fall was only part of a bigger battle between the forces of God and evil. 'We are fighting against the evil rulers of the unseen world, those mighty satanic beings and great evil princes of darkness who rule this world, and against huge numbers of wicked spirits in the spirit world.'[9]

## Suffering—God's passive role

God's relationship to suffering may be considered as both passive and active.

### *Why did God permit evil in the first place?*

Even though there is evidence that God did not directly design evil and that it came from a being opposed to Him, we are still left with a problem. If He is omnipotent, why did He allow it? If suffering is the result of man's choice, why did He make man able to choose? The author suggests that it was not because He does not care, but rather because He does, that He did so. God gave to man a free will. He is the only one of God's created beings that does not keep to the rules because he is the only one with power not to keep them. Without the power to choose, to obey or to disobey, to do good or to sin, to hate or to love, and above all to love God, he would not be a man, but a robot. A robot has no dignity. Love is surely man's highest attribute, and love, to be love, must be spontaneous and free. If man is to have the power to love, then he must also have the power 'not to love'. If man is to have freedom of choice then there must be at least two courses of action open to him.

God's gift of freewill to man gives an insight into the heart of a caring Creator. There must be a sense in which God needs man, He designed him for fellowship with Himself. He loves him with an everlasting love and longs for man's response to that love.

*But why does God allow suffering to go on?*

Surely, we ask, if God were a God of love He would not allow human suffering to go on! Would He not intervene to stop it? But we need to think carefully what it is we are expecting God to do. We are asking Him to negate the results of man's sin without removing the cause. This would mean the disruption of the laws of cause and effect. There are certain things that simply do not 'pay', certain actions which bring their own retribution, sins which bring their own punishment, and so I refrain from them. To remove human suffering would be to remove its limiting effect and unleash the ravages of sin, greed and cruelty. In fact man would surely destroy himself and society would cease to exist. Further, if God were to remove the ultimate in suffering, namely death, life as we know it now would become eternal and a worse hell could hardly be imagined.

Moreover, God knows that there is something worse than suffering and death, namely eternal separation and estrangement from Himself. In the medical sphere how many times have we wished that cancer were painful in its early stages! Just as physical pain may be beneficent because it points out a killing disease that can be cured, so human suffering in a wider sense points out the destructive nature of sin which by the grace of God and His action on our behalf can be cured before it is too late.

Most important of all, to ask God to remove suffering is to ask Him to change the essential nature of man and to remove his free will. To remove suffering means to remove the cause of suffering, namely sin, and therefore to remove man's power to sin and so his power to choose. But it is not only his freedom to sin that he would lose; but also his freedom to turn in repentance toward God and to choose the good. The Bible specifically states that this is one reason why God has not intervened to stop it all, 'He is waiting, for the good reason that He is not willing that any should perish, and He is giving more time for sinners to repent.'[10]

## Suffering—God's active role

So far we have suggested the possible reasons for God's allowing suffering in the world, and so have been considering His passive or permissive role. What of His positive action with regard to human suffering? This can conveniently be considered in two spheres, in the history of the human race, and in the lives of individuals.

### God's action—in history

Sometimes we hear the question asked 'Why does God stand by and watch human suffering?' Such a question needs to be answered, and any idea that God's attitude towards suffering is wholly passive resolutely refuted. The one thing that God has not done is to 'stand by'. He has been involved from the start and even before it, for in the Bible, the record of God's activity with regard to man, there are indications that His plans were ready before the moment of man's rebellion.[11] The explicit promise of God to act on behalf of fallen man is stated in Genesis 3:15. That promise is repeated and expanded in His word to the patriarchs and leaders of Israel, and prophesied in detail in such passages as Isaiah 53.

Throughout the pages of the Old Testament we see the long years of God's preparation of His people, His patience with their rebellion and obstinacy, and His perseverance in seeking lost mankind. But it is in the New Testament that we see the promise fulfilled in the coming of Jesus, for 'When the time had fully come God sent forth His Son, born of a woman, born under the law, to redeem those who were under the law, so that we might receive the adoption of sons.'[12] We need to notice that though He was the Son of God 'He became a human being[13] and it is in His dual nature that we begin to understand God's purpose. In His manhood He came to fulfil God's original purpose, He was the only man in whom God's image has remained wholly unspoiled. In His Godhead He came to redeem man who had lost that image and to restore it.

### Christ's attitude towards human suffering

In Christ's attitude to human suffering we see a perfect reflection of God's attitude since 'I and the Father are one'[14] and, 'Anyone who has seen Me has seen the Father.'[15] It is illuminating to read again the four Gospels with this in mind.

Firstly we see that Jesus was 'moved with compassion' not only to the point of tears but to the point of action. He knew the true nature of sympathy or 'suffering with'. To Him it was not a sterile offering of condolence, a means of avoiding the truth, evading the issue and sparing Himself; but a warm, deep love that issued in action on behalf of the sufferer. It was costly, 'healing power went out from Him',[16] and, in the presence of bereavement, 'He was moved with indignation and greatly troubled.'[17] There is no occasion recorded when He turned down a request for help. He exhausted Himself in the service of those who suffered so that He even slept through a storm on the lake. Moreover He was always 'on the side' of the sufferer, and never aggressive towards him as sometimes we are, almost blaming the patient for not responding to our treatment.

Secondly, He was able to deal with the results of man's wrong choices, namely disease, suffering and death. His power to heal was not selective. 'No matter what their diseases were . . . the touch of His hands healed every one.'[18] He was even Master of death itself, and at His command, Lazarus, dead for three days, rose up and came out of the tomb.[19]  The only people He could not help were those who were unaware that they were sick.[20]

And thirdly, He not only cured the results of the sins of mankind but He understood and dealt with its cause in the individual, often demonstrating the intimate association between physical cure and forgiveness. 'Now you are well' He said to the man crippled for thirty-eight years. 'Don't sin as you did before, or something even worse may happen to you.'[21]  'I have authority on earth to forgive sin . . . I'll prove it to you by healing this man.'[22]  On one occasion, too, He indicated publicly that suffering is the result of the devil's activity.  Healing the woman 'bent double' and unable to 'straighten herself' He spoke of the 'bondage in which Satan has held her for eighteen years'.[23]

*Christ's involvement in human suffering*

But Jesus did more than deal with human suffering as He met it, He Himself suffered with us.  He who was the God of heaven[24] submitted to the weakness and helplessness of the incarnation, and the rough and tumble and the frustrations of an earthly home.  He knew the struggle against poverty, and experienced the discomforts of hunger, thirst, weariness and homelessness.  He knew the heartache of utter loneliness and misunderstanding. He suffered the jealousies of those He had come to help and the tearing of His heart when His best gifts were thrown back by those He loved, and when He was rejected by those He was suffering so much to save.  At the end of it all He underwent the exquisite suffering of the Cross, the more acute because of the sensitivity of a mind and body unblunted by the ravages of sin

But He did even more than suffer with us, He suffered for us, and this surely is the ultimate proof of His caring.[25]  There was something unusual about His death. He shrank from it in the garden of Gethsemane, 'My soul is crushed with horror and sadness to the point of death . . . my Father, if it be possible, let this cup be taken away from me.'[26] He was desolated by His suffering on the Cross, 'My God, My God, why have you forsaken Me?'[27] Are we to believe that this was cowardice and lack of faith such as lesser men have not shown? Or was it that He was bearing what you and I can never bear, the burden of the sin of the world? Was it that God, who cannot allow sin in any form,[28] did indeed turn away from His only Son, since 'for our sake He made Him to be sin Who knew no sin, so that in Him we might become the righteousness of God?'[29] and that Jesus bore a separation from God that He had never known before, for your sake and mine, and that, most wonderful of all, He did it voluntarily because He loved us?[30]

God, by the Cross, took man's greatest tragedy and with it forged our salvation, so that now He can offer us forgiveness, a restored relationship with Himself and peace of heart in a society that knows no peace. He offers newness of life and a new dimension for living (in spite of the limitations of disease and deterioration) and a new horizon, a new perspective where death becomes an incident in a far bigger life, far from decaying with the years, becoming better and better as it blossoms into eternity.[31]

### God's action in the life of the individual

We may feel that it is all very well to talk of God's intervention in human history, but what about us and our patients? Is there any evidence that God cares about suffering in the lives of individuals? Once we have grasped the significance of what He did on the Cross, and why He did it, we have a new insight into His dealings with men. If He cared enough to die for me there must be some purpose in what He allows in my life, even if I cannot at first see it or understand it.

First we see that suffering causes us to think. The question 'why has this happened to me?' implies that we can understand it happening to others whom we regard as less deserving than ourselves. But when we consider the holiness of God and His standard for us, and then look at ourselves, we recognize that a more sensible question would be 'why has this not happened to me before?' Correct diagnosis is the first step towards cure, and to face the truth about ourselves heralds the dawn of a new hope. Just as pain points out a killing disease which can be cured, so suffering may point out that all is not well between us and God. The only people He cannot help are those who are unaware of their need.[32]

Secondly, suffering reminds us of the transitoriness of life, how short and futile it is. For 'we are but dust, and our days are few and brief, like grass, like flowers, blown by the wind and gone forever'.[33] Most of the things we seek give only fleeting pleasures and certainly cannot be taken with us beyond the grave. Moreover, it is one of our modern illusions that health is normal and ours by right. The fact is, however, that man's mortal life is running down all the time, and disease, degeneration and death are normal.

Thirdly, suffering often highlights a different quality of life, a new dimension of experience which could be ours, independent of circumstances. Often we have seen it in those who suffer most. For God can do something greater than save us from trouble, He can save us in it. We have no need to run away from suffering and to evade the issue. We have seen for ourselves people whose lives have been deep and serene, effective and worthwhile in spite of, and indeed because of, tremendous disability.

Lastly, suffering makes people think about what lies ahead. Is there a life after death? Is death the end? Questions like these are sometimes asked by the most unlikely patients when they really begin to face the issue of death.  They begin to wonder whether there is something worse than death, they begin to doubt, not if there is a heaven, but whether they will be adjudged worthy of it.  Yet, on the other hand we have seen some people die without fear, with their eyes on the distant horizon, upheld by a sure and certain hope, awaiting with glad expectancy the redemption of the body to a life without pain and sorrow.[34]  We have watched the manner of their dying and have seen that they have met face to face One Whom they already knew.  Such patients give us, as doctors, much cause to think in an age of medicine which has two obsessions.  One is that life in this world must be prolonged at all costs, even if it is not life but the process of dying that we prolong.  The other, in strange contradiction, is that all distress must be fully relieved even to the point of terminating life itself.

## Approaching the suffering and death of our patients

Having faced the principles underlying the problem of our approach to suffering and death, we find ourselves in a position to consider the questions that arise in our handling of our patients.  Our attitude at this point depends largely on our relationship to the truth.  Is not the Truth ultimately a *Person*, who holds our allegiance?[35]  Do we judge truth? or does Truth judge us?

Is it true that the doctor (any more than anyone else) knows when to lie?  To many medical people, it is undesirable that a patient be aware of his prognosis and of the incurability of his disease.  But to the Christian, who sees that disease and death are the symptoms of a broken relationship between God and the human race, and that by the grace of God that relationship can be restored in Christ, awareness of the temporariness of life might not be a disadvantage at all.  If there is something to be feared which is worse than death, namely eternal separation from God, then can it be helpful to deny the truth to the patient who deliberately asks to be told?  Doctors

75

who mislead their patients at this point would seem to take upon themselves a very heavy responsibility indeed.

Further, the patient who has been misled almost inevitably finds out the truth in the end. At this moment of realization he is in desperate need of someone to whom he can talk: not someone too closely involved as are his relatives, but someone he knows a little and can respect. He probably knows no Christian minister, and his thoughts naturally turn to his doctor. But the doctor who has lied has lost his respect, and is unlikely to be able to help him again. A Christian matron of a Terminal Home known for its happiness was asked her opinion in this matter. She replied, that those that did not yet know the truth and those already aware of it she could help; but those who had been misled were so embittered when they actually found out the truth, that no one was able to help them at all. On the grounds therefore of wisdom, quite apart from right, it would seem that patients' questions should be answered honestly.

There is a further point which deserves consideration. The policy often adopted of telling a husband of his wife's prognosis and refusing to tell the patient, puts a barrier between the two at a time when there should be no barrier. Indeed the barrier may be false, because it is often the case that both know the truth, but for the sake of the other they bear it alone. They deny themselves and each other the mutual support and comfort which is their right.

There remain many questions whose answers can only be dictated by individual circumstances and the growing experience of the doctor. Who should tell? How much to tell? When to tell? How to tell? Should the patient who doesn't ask ever be told? Or is the protective barrier the patient often puts around himself not for our breaking? While on some occasions it may be appropriate to refer the question to the doctor in charge of the case, there are often in ourselves attitudes which hold us back, which we wrongly attribute to our concern for the patient. We rightly dislike inflicting suffering yet are daily prepared to inflict suffering that a cure may be effected. Often we are really more concerned about the unpleasantness of the reaction on us, and the awkwardness for us of the situation which may result, rather than about the effect on the patient. We realize too, that to discuss so profound an issue with our patients takes time, imagination and costly involvement which we are not prepared to face, and so we try to keep our relationship superficial.

On the other hand, we sometimes speak purely to salve our own consciences and go away priding ourselves on having spoken the truth, yet leaving behind us chaos of thought and misery of spirit. To the Christian doctor and nurse, the privilege of talking over the future with a patient should surely be an opportunity to be prayed for, rather than an ordeal to be avoided. It would be well for many of us to consider the opportunities that are ours when our patients are not incurably ill, when much of their life is still before them, since the Bible reminds us that men 'through fear of death have been living all their lives as slaves to constant dread.[36]

For the Christian doctor there can be no question of Euthanasia, of assuming a God-like power of determining the moment of a patient's death. Yet we all know that pain-relieving drugs, used to the point of controlling pain, may well dull intellect and shorten life. Surely, the matter of motive is of importance here; our object must always be to save life, and to make that life of the highest quality possible in the circumstances. Yet even here we need to remember our limitations. We need more often to realize that all that medicine can do in the end is to push death further away and to make it easier. All too often however we manage to prolong the process of dying. Again, experience, compassion and a deepening understanding of the ways of God alone can teach us when to attempt radical treatment, and when to limit our treatment to palliation.   In any case, those of us to whom it falls to decide on the nature and extent of major surgical procedures, must rigorously resist the temptation to add one more case to our series, rather than to do that which we believe to be in the best interest of our particular patient.

We need always to retain an attitude of humility in these matters.   The problem of suffering is a mystery, and will remain so in this life.   Never let us speak as though we have got it 'tied up'.   Let us realize with gratitude that in our fight against suffering and death we are working together with God.   Jesus spoke of the woman who had been kept prisoner by Satan for eighteen long years[37] and death is after all 'the last enemy'.[38] Let us remember too, how great is our privilege in 'suffering with' our patients as they (and we) face the transitoriness of life, and the futility of much that it offers.

It is the people that we are and the Presence we manifest that determines our reactions to the problems our patients raise.   Moreover the extent to which we have faced these issues ourselves, and found their answers in the Lord Jesus Christ, will determine what questions are asked of us and what opportunities of witness are presented to us.   We can never push people into faith, we can only lead them where we have gone ourselves. We can never give them what we have not ourselves received.   And surely this is not a 'commodity', but a Person.   It is the Lord Jesus Christ alone Who can teach us, as we walk in daily contact with Him, how and to whom He would have us speak.

## References*

1 Genesis 1:31.
2 Genesis 1:27-30.
3 Genesis 3:10.
4 Genesis 3:12.
5 Genesis 3:16.
6 Genesis 3:17-19.
7 Genesis 3:6 R.S.V.
8 Genesis 3:1-5.
9 Ephesians 6:12.
10 2 Peter 3:9.
11 Revelation 13:8.
12 Galatians 4:4 R.S.V.
13 John 1:14, Hebrews 2:16.
14 John 10:30.
15 John 14:9.
16 Luke 6:19.
17 John 11:33.
18 Luke 4:40.
19 John 11:43,44.
20 Matthew 9:12.
21 John 5:14.
22 Matthew 9:2-7.
23 Luke 13:10-16.
24 Philippians 2:5-8.
25 John 15:13.
26 Matthew 26:38,39.
27 Matthew 27:46.
28 Habakkuk 1:13.
29 2 Corinthians 5:21 R.S.V.
30 John 10:18.
31 Proverbs 4:18.
32 Revelation 3:17,18.
33 Psalm 103:14-16.
34 Romans 8:23, Revelation 21:3-5.
35 John 14:6.
36 Hebrews 2:15.
37 Luke 13:16.
38 1 Corinthians 15:26.

*Unless otherwise stated the Biblical references are taken from the Living Bible.

## Further Reading

Twycross R. G. *The dying patient.* London: CMF Publications, 1975.

# 8 Miraculous healing

Vincent Edmunds

THERE is a continuing, or increasing, interest in the subject of Miraculous Healing. Two reasons stand out. In spite of the enormous progress made in the field of therapeutics in the past few decades, there are nevertheless large areas in medicine where the doctor can do little, or nothing, of curative value. It is, therefore, not surprising that in such circumstances some patients or their relatives, after taking second or maybe third opinions, turn in their distress for help to the paranormal or supernatural. Added to this there has been in recent years the widespread growth of the Charismatic Movement in all branches of the Church, with its special emphasis on spiritual gifts, including that of healing. Claims and counter-claims are made by Christian and non-Christian alike so that the seeker after truth is bewildered and does not know what to think or believe. Some go so far as to state that miraculous healing should be the normal experience of every truly committed Christian.

## Definitions

It is always good at the outset of any discussion to be certain how the subject is to be defined, and this is certainly necessary when reviewing miraculous healing. The Concise Oxford Dictionary describes miracle as 'a marvellous event due to some supernatural agency'. This provides a good working definition. And of course nowhere are such marvellous events better illustrated than in the varied miracles of Christ. These included acts of healing which were unique when compared with other contemporary methods of healing. A variety of diseases were cured, many of which would still today be considered as incurable; the cure was instantaneous (or almost so) in all cases; it was complete and lasting. Such miracles of healing were also performed by the Apostles during the first years of Church history. Having defined the subject, the question which is commonest today is, 'Do such healings in the New Testament meaning of the term occur today? If so, should we expect them as a regular feature of the Church's life?'

## Related topics

There are other matters which closely impinge upon miraculous healing – subjects such as 'spiritual', 'divine' and 'faith' healing. Though related, these adjectives are not the same as 'miraculous', since each emphasizes a different aspect of the subject, and some of these terms are more precisely definable than others. For instance 'spiritual' healing can mean healing by the power of the Holy Spirit, though equally well and frequently it is used, in public reporting, of healing by a spiritualist healer. For others, the words imply healing in the spiritual experience of the sufferer. Then 'divine' healing needs further definition, since all healing is fundamentally from God. We have still much to learn about the common healing processes, and the doctor much of the time remains a spectator, doing what he can to assist 'nature'. He often feels like the much quoted Ambroise Paré, the Huguenot surgeon, who said: 'I dressed the wounds; God healed them.' As for 'faith' healing – faith, while an important ingredient in some of them, was by no means invariably demonstrated in those who benefited from Christ's miracles of healing. Furthermore, when talking of faith, it is important to define the *object* in which, or in whom, the subject confides his trust. The object could be far from Christian. Indeed, it could be something quite nebulous.

Every clinician recognizes the importance of gaining the confidence (faith) and co-operation of his patient, if his treatment is going to meet with real success. This co-operation is indeed of great assistance, and accounts for much of the placebo effect of medication. In clinical trials of new medicines, up to 35 per cent of patients with organic disease will show some improvement on an inert preparation. This figure rises to over 40 per cent when the sufferer's disease is in the mind rather than the body. Patients are to some extent under their doctors' spell, but by the same token of course the patient who has no desire to recover and who refuses to co-operate, but turns his face to the wall, may soon expire in spite of his doctor's efforts on his behalf. This is part of the psychology of healing and an illustration of the place of faith in therapy.

Faith healing, then, can be a rather nebulous entity; but not so miraculous healing. Here attention is shifted from the operation of faith, though this may be an important ingredient, to the mechanism of healing. As we have already seen above, it is healing without resort to medical means in diseases which are often incurable. The recovery is also instantaneous, or almost so, complete and without relapse. To repeat the question, do such healings occur today? If they occur, then how often? Are we entitled to expect them as a regular feature of the Christian's experience? There are those who claim that this should indeed be the case, that there is a neglected spiritual gift which we should be seeking, and that there are those in this and other countries who are exercising it fruitfully.

## Healing activities

Claims of healings come from various parts of the world and also from specific healing centres. The best known of these is the Roman Catholic shrine at Lourdes in France. This little town has a normal population of 10,000, but in the months of April to October this is swollen by visitors to between 40,000 and 120,000. Many of these visitors will go to the famous grotto. Then, at Crowhurst in Sussex there is a less well-known, but similar, centre called the Home of Divine Healing. Also, at various times in different parts of the Mission Field claims of miraculous healing are made, e.g. in Southern Africa, South America and Indonesia to cite only a few.

The accounts make dramatic reading. Because the reports are so often given in popular terms there is difficulty in the substantiation of many of these claims.

Accurate medical evidence is usually sadly lacking. In 1973 in Dar-es-Salaam Cathedral in Tanzania a great many miraculous healings were said to have taken place. A variety of ailments including asthma, blindness, impotence and leprosy were mentioned as having been cured. However, an African doctor who knew the area well wrote: 'During my career in this country there have been many such reported healings, particularly in the areas on both sides of Lake Nyasa. All the outbreaks have followed the same pattern, i.e. tremendous popularity initially with thousands of people being attracted to the meetings, but with gradual thinning out of the attendances. When the popularity has waned, the outbreak and the organiser move to another area. My own impression is that there is nothing to these healings and that the initial popularity decreases as the actual results become known. I have not come across a single case of undoubted cure, proved by the clinical condition before and after the alleged healing.'

At Lourdes since 1958 there has been a Medical Bureau which investigates the claims of healing and only allows their registration as 'miraculous' if they meet certain standards of authentication. Many 'cures', of course, leave the town and never get investigated by the Bureau. It accepts as miraculous six to seven cases a year. This number should be seen in the light of the hundreds of thousands who visit the grotto. It seems in general that many claims of miraculous healing must be accepted with a respectful scepticism when they have not been scrutinized by someone with medical training, who is able to make a clinical assessment of the pathological state before and after the 'healing'.

## Medical aspects

The word 'miracle' is one which has become devalued. It is not always used with its original implications. 'My doctor says it was a miracle. He was amazed at the way I had recovered.' Perhaps it *was* a miracle. More likely, however, it was an unexpected improvement or recovery which had seemed to be highly unlikely at the time it occurred, but not impossible. Whenever attempts are made in all good faith to obtain clinical details and accurate diagnoses to substantiate claims of miraculous healing, such details are either not obtainable or the doctor is accused of lack of faith in presuming to ask for them. In practice, however, the Christian practitioner who is called upon to comment upon a claim to miraculous cure should not cease to use his intelligence and scientific training simply because he is confronted with the results of what is claimed as a supernatural intervention. Constant attempts have, therefore, been made by Christian doctors to collect and assess the medical details, but with singular lack of success.

When seeking such information we need to be aware of the many differing factors which are daily concerned in the progress and cure of disease. These include the influence of the emotions, the effect of suggestion, and the use of specific therapy. Even spontaneous remission of 'incurable' diseases may occasionally occur. Critical examination of the work of 'healers' shows that the majority of the 'cures' involve functional or non-organic diseases. In a large gathering met for a healing service emotional factors must be especially operative. A patient may as the result of an encounter with a healer, or attendance at a healing meeting, feel better in himself. These feelings may be engendered by the sympathy expressed by the healer or the 'aura' of his presence, or again the emotional influence of the meeting. A re-orientation of the patient's attitude to his disease may have a similar effect, that is, when perhaps he comes to accept his disability more philosophically and with less rebellion. (When this occurs in a Christian context, this is wholly good, and it is what Christian concern and care is all about – but it is not a 'miracle'.) Any, or all, of these benefits may be hailed as a 'cure' by the un-critical observer, including maybe the popular press.

## A BMA enquiry

In 1956, in reply to a request for information on super-natural healing from the Archbishops' Commission on Healing, the British Medical Association produced a Report[1] on an investigation conducted throughout the country. The report was sympathetically phrased, but it had to admit to no clear medical evidence in favour of miraculous healing. Closer investigation of claims had proved these to have arisen for several reasons – (1) There had been a mistake in diagnosis. (How easy it is to make a diagnostic mistake on occasions, especially if there is no supporting histology available!) (2) There were mistakes in prognosis. Every doctor knows that one of the most difficult things in medicine is to say just how long a patient will survive in a certain situation. (3) There were cases where there had been temporary alleviation of pain and freedom from symptoms, e.g. by hypnotic suggestion. (4) There were remissions in the disease process. These are well recognized as occurring from time to time in diseases such as multiple sclerosis.

(5) Then there were a few spontaneous cures. These have been recorded in the literature even, albeit rarely, in all forms of cancer. There has been no suggestion that non-orthodox measures have been adopted in these cases. (6) There were also found numerous cases in which the pursuit of ordinary medical treatment had continued at the same time as attendance at a healing centre. To this could be added the delayed beneficial effects of treatment previously administered, particularly in the case of radiotherapy and chemotherapy – the planned improvement coinciding with a visit to a healer.

Space does not permit a more detailed discussion of individual claims. Suffice it to say that investigations, both before and since the BMA report, have – with a very few notable exceptions – failed to find medical evidence to support extensive claims of miraculous healing. Dr. Arthur Hill, a Canadian physician, in 1954 wrote in a booklet entitled *Divine Healing*:[2] 'For 20 years I have been tracking down cases such as these. In the few where medical reports are actually available, the result has always been the same – no miraculous cure.'

## Miracles in scripture

Miraculous activity is found recorded in Scripture not as a continuous happening but as sporadic occurrences. These events were almost invariably related to specific historical events or periods. In the Old Testament the lives of Moses, Elijah and Elisha were particularly associated with miracles of several different types. Those were times of spiritual re-awakening and special revelation after periods of apostasy. Jehovah used this method to authenticate his chosen leaders. The same may be said of Christ's miracles, particularly those of healing. Compassion undoubtedly prompted many of these. Nevertheless the clear inference from Scripture is that they were intended to serve a more specific purpose, which was to convince the Jews that the promised and long expected Messiah had now come. The clearest indication of this was on the occasion when John the Baptist[3] sent messengers from his prison cell to enquire whether Jesus was indeed the Christ. The reply was not a reasoned argument, but a practical demonstration of His miraculous powers.

Similarly, the powers delegated to the Apostles served to authenticate their message before their opponents in Israel and to establish the infant Church. Healing campaigns such as occur today were not part of the New Testament picture. Christ's healings were not organized; they were incidental; supporting, but subordinate, to His *teaching*. Here we find Him moving to other towns so that He might *teach* there also. There we find Him urging secrecy upon those whom He has healed. Surely this was so that He might avoid becoming known simply as a healer and miracle-worker rather than as a teacher. His healings appear sometimes to have been provocative. Was His use of the Sabbath Day for this purpose coincidental or intentional? It never failed to anger His hypocritical critics.

## The experience of the Apostles

But what of such verses as 1 Corinthians 12:9,28-30 and James 5:14,15? Detailed analysis and comment are precluded here. In the former, however, Paul is speaking of specific gifts given by the Spirit to selected individuals. All believers have their gift, or gifts. They are distributed in a sovereign manner at the Holy Spirit's discretion and presumably may equally well be withdrawn in similar manner. They are for the common good. Paul found the Corinthian Church lacking in spirituality (1 Corinthians 1 to 3). Yet they eagerly ask him questions about spiritual gifts. He outlines them but tries to encourage a balanced view of them and a true perspective. He indicates that love is better than all the gifts, including that of 'languages' (1 Corinthians 13:1). Furthermore, the ability to communicate the

Gospel is crucial and to be desired above that of speaking in languages (1 Corinthians 14:5).

Most of the Nineteenth Century expositors argued that the gift of healing died out with the establishment of the early Church. Certainly no reference is made to healing in Ephesians 4:11 or Romans 12:6-8. Neither is there mention of it in the latest Epistles of the New Testament – Pastoral Epistles – which would give some support to this view. There is, too, much evidence to indicate that the Apostles and their fellow-workers did not avail themselves of supernatural healing if such were readily available. The fact that Paul with his thorn in the flesh,[4] Timothy[5] with his gastric upsets, together with Epaphroditus[6] and Trophimus,[7] found no easy cure for their illnesses shows that miraculous healing of believers was not invariable, or to be taken for granted.

## The Epistle of James

Such considerations help to put James 5:14,15 into proper perspective. A full discussion is beyond the scope of this article and the interested reader should consult such authorities as Prof. Tasker,[8] or the Memorandum published by the CMF.[9] It is good, however, to have these verses in perspective. Taking the balance of Scripture is particularly important here since we appear to have a definite instruction concerning how we should proceed in the event of illness. In brief, these verses, if taken at their face value, would mean that no Christian need ever die. He must simply, when in need, call on the elders of the Church who will pray for him for recovery, which will ensue. Since this is patently untrue, what do they mean?

1. It is to be noted that this is addressed to *believers* who are sick. They are advised – not to attend a healing service – but to call on the elders. It is a private affair, not a public meeting.
2. The place of oil is open to discussion and some hold that the Greek would indicate a form of therapy

rather than simply symbolic anointing. In other words, the proper use of medical means is not precluded, but rather encouraged.

3. Prayer is offered in faith for the sick person and the answer, as with all prayer, is in God's hands. We cannot indicate what He in His sovereign mercy will do, but only pray that His will may be done.

4. The phrase concerning 'raising up' referred to in verse 15 is, in the context, equivocal. It could indicate the restoration of bodily health. Equally, however, it could contain a promise of future resurrection life. While these verses would not appear in any way to contain a blue-print for healing, the instruction is nevertheless sometimes practised by devout Christians in times of severe illness. As such it is a source of encouragement and spiritual support to both the sick and their relatives.

## Recapitulation

Our review of the subject of 'Miraculous Healing' would indicate that the types of miraculous healing described in the Bible were largely peculiar to the time of Christ, His apostles and the early church. If such occur today in that form then, according to the medical evidence, they seem to do so extremely rarely. Having stated this, however, we must reiterate that God is Sovereign in these things and we admit to, and believe, in the possibility of such an occurrence if the circumstances were such that it was God's will. Here again, it would be for Him to decide the occasion and the circumstances. But, as in the early church, authentication of the messenger, or his message, in an area of heathendom or an era of apostasy, might be the Holy Spirit's reason for a further outpouring of miraculous activity, including miraculous healing.

## Health and wholeness

While our present remit is 'miraculous healing' it is

important for us to view it in its full context. The word 'healing' has a wide connotation in modern Christian thought and writing, particularly from charismatic believers. Physical healing is certainly involved but thinking goes far beyond this to include the mending of personal relationships, both within and outside marriage, and more fundamentally to the forgiveness of sin. That such events are one kind of 'healing' in a person's life cannot be disputed; that they are valuable and necessary goes without saying; but they are not 'miraculous healing' as we have been discussing it. To give an example – Francis McNutt[10] an American Roman Catholic priest, who has written what is acknowledged to be one of the best books on healing from the charismatic standpoint, recognizes healing under *four* separate headings, only one of which is of organic disease. They are: (1) Moral sickness resulting from personal sin. (2) Emotional sickness caused by anxiety and emotional hurts of our past. (3) Physical sickness caused by disease or accident. (4) Any of the above caused by demonic oppression.

## A healing ministry

He writes well, enthusiastically and persuasively, but it is apparent that the healing of *physical* disease is but a small part of what he regards as Christian healing, or what others might refer to as the 'Church's ministry of healing'. So far as the physical healings are concerned, McNutt is aware of some of the problems of reporting that we have reviewed here, but he is in the main convinced of their genuineness. Medical comment on the pathology involved is, however, largely lacking.

McNutt presents a view of 'healing' which is widely held in the Church today. It stretches from the healing of structural disease on the one hand, through psychosomatic illness to frankly emotional and spiritual disturbances on the other. While not questioning the sincerity of its proponents, it is not always easy to say when the claimed healings have been due to a genuine encounter with God, and when there has been little more than an emotional 'shot in the arm', resulting from contact with a Christian counsellor. The value of the work undertaken in the name of 'Christian healing' is beyond question, but many feel that to call it by such a name is to add confusion to what is already a bewildering subject.

## Prayer – a science?

To return briefly to McNutt. He does raise a disturbing issue when he quotes (page 31) efforts to demonstrate scientifically the power of prayer. 'Rev. Franklin Loehr reports in his book *The Power of Prayer on Plants*, the results of 156 persons praying in 700 unit experiments using more than 27,000 seeds and seedlings . . . and achieving 52.71% growth advantage for prayer seedlings.' He further quotes – 'Dr. Bernard Grad tested the speed with which wounds heal in mice . . .' under the influence of the laying on of hands.

The mind boggles. The possibilities for the Christian gardener seem endless! We must not pursue this line too far for it opens up many questions if prayer to God does actually influence such natural phenomena in the manner described. The danger which we should recognize is – assuming, of course, that it is God and not some other spiritual power who is responsible for these biological happenings – that we shall tend to reduce and to view the power of God as just another *form of therapy*. As much as to say 'Medicine and Surgery have been tried with very little success, now what about prayer?' It is as though man has discovered a trigger which he only has to press for seeds to grow better, mice to heal quicker and presumably man also to recover from all his illnesses. To be fair to McNutt he simply quotes these experiments, but does not develop an argument from them. However, the basic thought described seems to be there and he seems to be in agreement with it. God, however, cannot be manipulated. Furthermore, He is not just another therapeutic tool to be wielded where necessary.

## The basic need

There is also a danger here of getting man's true needs into their wrong order – in other words a reversed perspective. For whatever man's physical state or disability, his basic need still remains forgiveness and spiritual regeneration, and not physical healing. It cannot, of course, be denied that Christ did on occasion forgive and heal at one and the same time. Such occurred for instance when the paralytic was brought to Him by his friends. Before acting, however, Jesus made the point firstly that forgiveness and healing are alike humanly impossible, and secondly that to God forgiveness is the prime consideration, physical needs being secondary.[11]

Arising from these, and similar passages in the Gospels, some would claim that Christ's healing was always a *complete* recovery of the person – body, mind and spirit. The natural sequel to such thinking is to argue that new-birth and forgiveness should bring '*wholeness*' to each one of us. It should be noted, however, that the disputed word 'whole' used in the Authorized Version has in the Greek text a purely physical context and did not carry any suggestion of spiritual renewal. This is made clear when a more modern translation is consulted. The Revised Standard Version, for example, uses expressions such as 'made well'[12] and 'well'[13] which are nearer to current usage and clearly indicate bodily healing. The New Birth is a spiritual experience and should be seen as such. It must be admitted that the radical changes in thought and life style which often accompany Christian conversion may lead to an all round improvement in health and physical wellbeing. This is a bonus when it occurs, but is not an inevitable outcome, any more than it was the reason for the conversion experience in the first instance.

## Other misapprehensions

The confusion of sickness and sin which has been referred to above usually seems to arise from a wrong understanding of Christ's redemptive work. The death of Christ, it is sometimes claimed, gives the believer 'a right' to healing and health. Superficial study of a few verses in Scripture might seem to give some support to this view. However, the weight of evidence in Scripture as a whole points to the fact that, although the Christian's redemption has already been completed, it will not in a physical sense be perfected in this life. In the same way that he finds himself burdened by his old nature, through which Satan seeks to weaken him and lead him astray, so also the believer continues to experience the frailty of his mortal body. Paul put it very clearly when he wrote we 'groan within ourselves, waiting for the adoption, to wit, the redemption of our bodies'.[14] Suffering in some shape or form will continue to be the Christian's lot until that day of final redemption, and Paul knew this only too well.[14] There is nothing to suggest that in this respect the Christian will fare any differently from the rest of mankind. No special favours or treatment are promised or indicated.

## Conclusions

At the outset mention was made of those who in desperation turn to 'healers' (of various types and backgrounds) in search of relief from a mortal or painful disease. Many are disappointed following their contact with such a 'healer'. For to their pain and suffering comes the additional distress that for some reason they have not been healed. 'Was it lack of faith?' they ask. Have their friends let them down? Should they all have prayed harder? Has God rejected their prayers? These and other thoughts torture their minds. A whole cycle of needless distress and mental anguish can be set in motion by those who make over enthusiastic, extravagant and unwarranted claims for healing.

As doctors we cannot admit to any special theological insights into the question of 'miraculous healing'. But we can claim, by virtue of our training and experience, to be able to diagnose organic disease and to recognize its healing and cure. This is our special responsibility when claims of healing are made. Their genuineness can thus be properly attested; the spurious and frankly phoney can also be recognized and exposed.

We have indicated above how much of the current interest in healing rests upon basic misconceptions concerning such things as health and wholeness, redemption and the reason for Christ's miracles. We could add to these further contemporary erroneous ideas concerning the nature of healing and about the purpose of suffering, which we have not touched upon. The fact is that numerous sympathetic and careful observers have been unable to find much evidence that 'miraculous healing' (in the New Testament sense) occurs today, though Christians must be open to its possibility. Yet, once a true Scriptural perspective has been achieved in these matters, the desire for sudden 'miraculous' intervention of the kind found in the Gospels largely disappears.

**References**

[1] *Divine Healing and Co-operation between doctors and clergy.* London: British Medical Association, 1956.
[2] Hill A. C. *Divine Healing.* Radio Gospel Fellowship, 1954.
[3] Luke 7:19-23.
[4] 2 Corinthians 12:7.
[5] 1 Timothy 5:23.
[6] Philippians 2:27.
[7] 2 Timothy 4:20.
[8] Tasker R. V. G. *Commentary on the Epistle of James.* London: Tyndale Press, 1956.
[9] Edmunds V., Scorer G. *Some thoughts on faith healing.* 3rd Ed. London: CMF Publications, 1979.
[10] McNutt F. *Healing.* Indiana, Ave Maria Press, 1974.
[11] Luke 5:20-24.
[12] Mark 5:34.
[13] Matthew 9:12.
[14] Romans 8:23.

**Further Reading**

Scorer C. G. *Healing: Biblical, medical and pastoral.* London: CMF Publications, 1979.

# 9  Medical treatment
## Duncan Vere

This topic may be divided into four parts:

(i) conventional treatment for physical or mental disorders; (ii) preventive treatment; (iii) experimental treatment; (iv) the use of some treatments where there is little or no disease.

## Conventional treatment

By conventional treatment is meant the common objective of restoring the abnormal, or diseased, person towards health.  It may have two aims: first the correction of abnormalities and then the relief of symptoms which they cause.  Often a third aim is to relieve the anxiety, or mental distress, caused by a disease. Whether only one, or more, of these purposes is followed, it should be done only in the patient's interest.  It must not be in the interests of the doctor, nor of any other person, unless the patient agrees to this knowingly and freely. At all times, whatever is done should conform to the best current medical practice.  Other types of treatment would be 'experimental', and will be discussed later.

Unfortunately, mistakes are sometimes made in attempts to treat patients and much disappointment and, indeed, illness may result.  Such mistakes may be purely technical – for example, errors of dose, of formulation and of the route of administration. More common and damaging is failure to be aware of, and understand, the signs and mechanisms of adverse drug reactions and interactions. The majority of mistakes, however, seem to occur through a faulty planning of the treatment, and by failing to explain to patients, and to check that they have understood, how a treatment should be applied. The essential *aim* is often overlooked or misunderstood.

Modern drugs are so powerful that doctors are tempted to imagine that they can end a number of diseases as if by magic. It is significant that the meaning of 'cure' has changed its meaning with the centuries to meet this idea. It originally meant 'to care for', in modern times it has come to mean 'to restore completely'. It is highly important to realize that all we can do is to assist the processes of natural recovery, not create it. Natural recovery may become complete, but it is not our remedies which will have achieved this. This is where Christian insights come in, for recovery is seen as God's gift and a part of life which is itself His gift. The doctor should retain a proper humility and 'creatureliness' before such facts, not assume the Creator's role in his imagination. This, of course, runs counter to humanist opinion about man's achievements.

A sound plan of treatment must be followed step by step. Mistakes must be noted if, and as, they occur. All really successful treatments begin with wise planning before any drugs have been taken by the patient. For example, wherever possible some *measurements* of the severity of the disease, however simple, should be obtained. It may be, for example, the measurement of the haemoglobin in iron deficiency, or grip-strength in rheumatoid conditions. Or a chart may be kept by the patient of the frequency of migraine. Such an approach is not meddlesome, or 'experimental', medicine. It is just ordinary common sense, for if one does not know how big something is before attempting to reduce it, how will one ever know wnether treatment has succeeded? The only doctors who have no need to measure are those who '*know*' that their treatments are always a success!

Then there is a choice of a remedy. We must sometimes remind ourselves that 'nothing' is a very useful drug. It is safe, costs nothing and is always available! Many drugs are given needlessly and many prescriptions are written almost by conditioned reflex. The mere existence of an abnormality does not necessarily prove that it should immediately be corrected. One particularly stupid reason for needless prescribing is the 'drug for the disease' mentality. Unhappily it is encouraged by some of the drug firms' advertisements. This is the attitude which says, 'If the disease is X, then the drug is Y.' A particularly banal example of such an attitude was an American advertisement of some years back. It showed a hand raised, with fingers on the pulse and the caption 'Slow it with reserpine'! It has been shown in a series of careful studies that a doctor's personal approach and care are as effective as drug treatment in helping sufferers from rheumatic diseases, or even in anaesthetic practice as premedication before anaesthesia. The only way to offset these faults is to begin to retrain society – patients *and* doctors – to accept that tablets are not a prerequisite in all therapy.

Before a drug is chosen (or an operation performed), a profit and loss account should be drawn up on the patient's behalf. It should take in the likely benefits, the risks, the costs and the patient's social and mental resources. Large numbers of prescribed treatments are too complex for the patient to follow. Drugs are often taken in ways which were never intended by the doctor. Particular care is needed with newly introduced remedies. Their profits often loom larger than their still uncertain risks.

There is also the highly difficult issue of which name to use, official or brand. Brand names have the advantage of simplicity and security. They describe drugs briefly and reveal their origin. This means that, should an accident ensue, the patient knows which company to sue! But brand names also obscure the chemical identity of drugs, and are often a device used by manufacturers to secure the profits from their drugs after the patent has lapsed. The cost of some, but not most, branded products far exceeds that of the un-branded or 'generic' drug. And it is impossible to learn clinical pharmacology without understanding the properties shared by drugs within each class of compounds; these classes can only be remembered simply by using approved names.

Particular thought should always be given before introducing a drug of potential dependence. Ever since barbiturates were rightly ousted by benzodiazepines, there have still been large numbers of unhappy, middle-aged people who seem unable to adjust to a changing life style and take to psychotropic drugs – alcohol, tricyclic antidepressants, tranquillizers and hypnotics. They really need advice and care, but have been conditioned by their doctors to ask for tablets instead. A newer problem is that many modern remedies involve taking over the control of a homeostatic system. Gone are the days when a fortnight's tablets might be 'tried'. Today tumours can be controlled by carefully regulated, continued therapy. Control of blood pressure, of endocrine functions and of excretion by dialysis are other examples. This complex and demanding type of remedy is better not begun if it cannot be sustained.

Before beginning any treatment it is always wise to ask how the results will be followed up. How and when should it be stopped? Many a doctor begins treatment without asking himself this question, which is like taking a car on to the road without steering or brakes.

Stopping treatment is particularly important, and difficult. Those who believe that their remedy is essential to the patient's life and wellbeing can never bring themselves to stop it. It is amazing how often, when someone else stops it, there is no apparent change for the worse! Many emotions surround the discontinuation of drugs. Anyone who has good grounds for thinking that his remedy is not helping a patient not only may, but should, stop it. This has sometimes been criticized as 'euthanasia', if it is thought that a life endangering illness is being held in check by the drugs. However, things are not so simple. Elderly people sometimes improve remarkably after an antibiotic has been withdrawn, perhaps because undetected superinfection with resistant germs had supplanted the initial invaders.

To withdraw a regime which is probably sustaining life is, of course, tantamount to damaging the patient. But it is not always certain whether the remedy is helping or harming. Then it is better to withdraw it and act on the information so gained. It is also sometimes said that withdrawing treatment removes the patient's hope. This need not be the case. A most valuable distinction has been suggested between 'treatment' and 'care'. Care is all that is not aimed at specific reversal of the disease, that is, symptomatic relief, skilled nursing and nutrition. This should never be withdrawn. (When unconscious, patients become harder to nurse if they are not nourished.) But elaborate and unnecessary drug regimes can and should be withdrawn, when progressive deterioration, often with multiple system failure, sets in. It follows that we should never say to a patient or his relatives that nothing can be done. This is the ultimate medical rejection. Care can *always* be given, and patients need reassurance to this effect.

The doctor's real dilemma is that there is no way to predict the outcome of treatment for an individual. Controlled trials and surveys help to provide probability estimates that a treatment will have, say, a 75 per cent chance of inproving disease X in the group of all of those who suffer from X. But this can never foretell whether

Mr. Y or Miss Z will be helped or harmed by it or by its withdrawal. This can only be established by trying the treatment. It goes without saying that doctors should observe the effects of what they try. Medical mishaps can often be averted by shrewd observation of the early stages of treatment effects.

Careless renewal of treatment is as bad as careless withdrawal. It is so easy for prescriptions to be renewed automatically, particularly when a new doctor takes over a case. It is equally easy for useful drugs to be forgotten and omitted. In summary, then, the aim is to use treatments compassionately, for the patient's natural recovery, wherever the likely benefits exceed the probable loss.

## Preventive treatment

Preventive treatment, or prophylaxis, is a relatively neglected method to attain positive health. It should gain renewed importance from the community health emphasis of the reorganizing health service. Public attitudes to prevention in Britain are curiously ambivalent, as the controversy over fluoridation of water supplies shows. It is indeed odd that families whose children are deemed to have been damaged by certain drugs are to be compensated but not those with children damaged by other therapeutic agents.

There is still a great deal of preventive medicine to be done. Even were there only a little truth in the 'bran story' the savings to the NHS from effective long term use of high fibre diets could be enormous. Looked at across the world, the lack of effective disease prevention is an international disaster. Countries which have relaxed their vigilance in preventing malaria, cholera and schistosomiasis are now reaping a pitiful harvest. This is strictly not medical treatment, but environmental prevention, unless one counts the cultivation of positive attitudes towards health as an aspect of preventive medicine. But it seems likely that a good deal of heart disease, hypertension, bronchitis, lung cancer and liver disease in developed countries could be prevented by modest dietary changes combined with moderation in the use of tobacco and alcohol. Indeed the incidence of heart attacks in North America is already showing a downward trend for no known cause other than changed attitudes to diet, exercise and tobacco.

## Experimental treatment

In a sense each treatment is an experiment, for its outcome can never be wholly foreseen. However, in a more precise sense all new remedies should be validated by adequate clinical experimental tests. Otherwise how would anyone be sure of their advantages? To say that 'a drug such as penicillin needed no controlled trial to prove its worth' is pointless. Even if the statement were true of penicillin, there are few drugs which can match its efficacy. Most need thorough trials to show their worth. It is an ethical obligation for any doctor who hopes to try a novel remedy to do so only in circumstances which will yield a clear, comparative result.

Placebos are legitimate treatments in such trials, provided that there is still doubt as to whether the remedy is, or is not, better than nothing. The doubts should include those of doctors other than the investigator. This is the principle behind local ethics committees to which all proposed new treatments should now be submitted in the British Isles. Trials are best conducted with several independent persons 'in the know' besides the investigator himself. The reason is that an individual can begin to believe in a treatment which he has developed long before anyone else would give it credit. The choice of a placebo depends also upon several other factors. For example, it may be correct to use placebos in disorders which do not endanger life or limb, or which cause little suffering. Examples might be trials of remedies for the common cold or migraine. By contrast, an anti-tumour drug or an antibiotic should not be compared with a placebo in otherwise similar situations.

If it is known that an effective remedy exists against serious disorders, however poorly effective it may be, then comparisons should be made against that remedy. A placebo should not be used.

## Treatment not essential to correct or prevent disease

Treatment may sometimes be carried out where there is no disease. Such a concept may seem astonishing at first sight, but in this century, this form of treatment has grown steadily and in practice continues to do so. C. G. Scorer has recently drawn attention to this new development. The position is that whereas conventional therapy restores the abnormal towards health, and preventive therapy modifies the normal so as to avert disease, there is a third area of choice. What of the actress who wants the shape of her nose changed to suit her performance? Or what of the 'pill' which prevents normal pregnancies, or the operation of vasectomy which alters normal structures with similar intent? Still more, what of abortion which destroys a normal, potential individual? Or the transsexualist demanding surgery, or the person who takes drugs to modify his conscious experience, or simply to assuage insecurity through a drug habit? In one sense these may be directed against disease, or towards its prevention, but it is so in a rather devious sense. The magnitude of the intervention often grossly outweighs the disorder. Often pleasure would seem to be the stronger reason for using (or abusing) remedies in such ways.

It is in this growing area that Christians are most likely to find themselves differing more and more from their fellow men. This is because they have a distinctive view of responsibility for life. They also have a concept of a divine purpose in man's nature which is foreign to others. Pleasure is not, for them, the highest good, although relief of suffering is a most proper object of compassion. They do not accept that what exists is necessarily good; but they do not feel it right to pursue a policy of change just because the possibility is there. In other words, 'feasibility' is not by itself a justification for any new intervention into human physiology. We should not, of course, be opposed to possible progress in new directions as a matter of principle. Many really good future advances will come, and must be 'received with thanksgiving'. But Christians will always want to ask searching questions about the purpose and benefits of each advance, and whether or not it fits into God's revealed views concerning the nature of Man.

## Further Reading

Vale J. A. The use and misuse of drugs. In, *Decision making in medicine: the practice of its ethics*. Ed. Scorer G, Wing A. London: Edward Arnold, 1979.

## 10 Research on patients

Ian Gordon-Smith

CLINICAL medicine, especially in the larger teaching hospitals, is increasingly supporting numbers of research workers whose primary interest is the extension of medical knowledge. To many people the idea of carrying out experiments on patients, even under the cloak of such phrases as 'controlled trial', 'clinical study' or 'additional investigations', undermines the whole foundation of the practice of medicine, based as it is on mutual trust between the doctor and his patient. As Sir William Heneage Ogilvie has written, 'experimental medicine . . . is capable of destroying in our minds the old faith that we the doctors are the servants of the patients whom we have undertaken to care for and, in the minds of the patients, the complete trust that they can place their lives, or the lives of their loved ones, in our care'.[1] Not only is the doctor-patient relationship threatened by medical research, but the patient himself may be exposed to discomfort and potential danger by the widening variety of ingenious instruments and techniques which allow visualization, measurement and biopsy of internal organs. Therefore it is vital to restate the grounds on which experiments on patients may be justified, the preconditions which must be fulfilled, and the ethical standards and motives which should influence the investigator.

## The role of clinical research

It has become axiomatic that any new method of investigation or treatment must be exhaustively tested and proved to be both safe and of value before it is applied in patients. This approach has come about as a consequence of several therapeutic misadventures which occurred because a new drug, e.g. thalidomide, or a new operation, e.g. Judet's hip replacement, was introduced on a large scale without proper preliminary studies in either animals or man. In fact many initial experiments may perfectly well be carried out in laboratory animals, notable examples being in the field of immunology and transplant surgery. However the whole process of the scientific method – observation leading to hypothesis, subsequently tested by experiment – applies not only to the laboratory model but also to the hospital patient, and the hypotheses tested in animal experiments have of necessity to be confirmed in man. An isotope which can be used to reveal venous thrombi in rabbits will probably be of value in the detection of deep vein thrombosis in postoperative patients, but a study in such patients will be necessary to prove this proposition. Similarly gastric ulceration in man may be preventable by a drug which protects rats against ulcer formation, but the inference cannot be made with certainty. Mice are not men and direct transfer of conclusions from the animal to man is not valid.

A particular problem in modern medicine is the profusion of new diagnostic and therapeutic techniques, and the energy with which these techniques are promoted. Clinical science fails unless the vigour of the promoter is matched by the rigour of the researcher. The methods by which innovations in medicine are assessed vary; but the controlled clinical trial has become established as one means. Doubtless few would query the ethics of performing a trial in which a potentially better drug is compared with an older but widely used compound. The advantages of this situation are obvious both for the patient and the doctor. However, objections may be raised when patients are asked to be willing to act as controls. Recently, for example, in patients with ulcerative colitis, active salazopyrin was compared with a dummy tablet. In this study the intention was to distinguish between any specific properties of the active drug and its placebo effects. Such a trial could be justified on the grounds that the patients included did not require any more therapy than the salazopyrin and this drug was itself of uncertain benefit. But clearly when the patient is in need of effective treatment and an agent is available which is known to be efficacious against his disease, then this agent and not an inert substance should be prescribed. However, when no such established therapy is available it is legitimate to compare the effects of a potentially valuable compound with a control or placebo group, always providing the patient's informed consent has been obtained prior to his inclusion in the trial. In this way the value of new approaches to diagnosis and therapy may be measured objectively and submitted to statistical analysis.

## Risks to the patient

Almost every action taken by a doctor in the process of relief of suffering is experimentation, although of an easily justifiable kind. This is true particularly in the context of the individual patient. Statistical analysis of previous research may indicate that 60 per cent of patients do well with one treatment, while 40 per cent respond better with another regimen. What the statistics cannot reveal is which therapy will be of greater benefit in this particular patient. The onus is upon the doctor to make this decision and the fact that the patient has placed himself in the doctor's hands implies consent to this process. Consequently, patients often find themselves to have been part of a research study although at the time they may have been ignorant that the study was in progress and their consent to inclusion was not sought. This circumstance is a common one, justified by the clinician on the grounds that no one type of diagnostic procedure or treatment has been proved to be superior to all others in the management of a particular disease. Studies of this nature are constantly in progress in most academic units, as for example in the random allocation of patients with breast cancer of equivalent clinical stage to treatment by simple or radical mastectomy, with or without radiotherapy. The patient can neither be held to be at increased risk by such random allocation nor can her consent reasonably be sought, for the simple reason that the doctor conducting the study does not know himself which regimen will ultimately be preferred.

The situation becomes much more complex and ethically problematical when the acts of the doctor are directed not to the benefit of the patient present but towards patients in general. Where the patient himself stands to gain from investigations performed, some risks are acceptable when weighed against the likely rewards. If, on the other hand, the patient will receive no advantage himself, but is merely contributing towards the welfare of future patients, any significant risk is only permissible provided the subject is himself able to appreciate the hazards and to give his assent without coercion.

Unfortunately, the concern for the patient's welfare and integrity has not always been upheld by clinical research workers in the way that respect for the individual dictates. Pappworth, in his startling book *Human Guinea Pigs*, cited many examples where patients had been exposed to considerable risks in investigations unrelated to their immediate problem. In many instances no evidence was available to state whether the patients knew the purpose of the investigations and had consented to them, or merely had believed them to be part of the management of their condition. Thus a group of doctors carried out coronary artery catheterization on fifty conscious exercising patients, half of whom suffered from coronary disease, but the other half acted as control patients of whom no details were given in the report of the results.[2] Experiments of this type could only be regarded as morally justified if the patients had been able to provide 'fully informed consent', a phrase with so many subissues that it requires further discussion.

## 'Fully informed consent'

Informing a patient as to the nature of a research project and obtaining his consent without pressurizing him is a very sensitive matter. 'It requires profound thought and consideration on the part of the physician for the complexities of medicine are in some cases so great it is not reasonable to expect that the patient can be adequately informed as to the full implications of what his consent means. His trust in the physician may lead him too easily to say "yes".'[3] Nevertheless, an effort has to be made to communicate the nature of the experimental procedure to the patient. He should know what risk he runs as the subject of research. Although the junior resident doctor and the clinical student are unlikely to have to carry out research procedures beyond the simple obtaining of specimens, doctors have a duty to ensure that patients in their care are aware that they are taking part in a research project and that they understand what is involved.

The question remains concerning the extent to which the patient should be informed of potential dangers. What constitutes full information? 'All experiments involve some risk. It may be an infinitesimally small one but it is always there.'[4] This being so, is every conceivable hazard to be communicated to the patient? Such a policy, though superficially correct and honest is clearly impracticable and would be likely to result in many subjects opting out of legitimate and valuable studies or becoming reluctant and apprehensive participants. Obviously the expected discomforts and effects of an investigation should be disclosed. A patient about to receive isotopically labelled human fibrinogen could reasonably anticipate that the nature of the radioactivity, its probable fate and the means of obviating any ill effects would be explained to him. On the other hand the very remote possibility that the fibrinogen might transmit the hepatitis virus would not normally be mentioned, being an almost unknown event with recent fibrinogen preparations, although still theoretically possible. This is only one example, but the issue of what to tell the subject for study recurs with every project undertaken.

Once informed as to the nature of the study the patient must be totally free either to agree to his inclusion or to opt out without feeling that if he elects for the latter course he will be receiving thereafter less of the doctor's interest and attention. The practising Christian has the golden rule first laid down by Christ to guide him – 'Whatever you wish that men would do to you, do so to them.'[5] Working in the light of this principle the doctor will never actively deceive his patients in order to secure their co-operation, and will place the interests of individual patients in his care above his own desire for additional clinical information.

## Motives in research

Sir Isaac Newton once described his discoveries as 'thinking God's thoughts after Him'. This is an apt definition of the revelations of science. The Christian view of the world created and sustained by an omniscient God leads naturally to a desire to unravel the intricacies of the living world. After the Reformation men of dynamic Christian faith were in the vanguard of scientific advance. Among these in the Nineteenth Century were Joseph Lister who developed antiseptic surgery and James Simpson who introduced chloroform anaesthesia into obstetrics. Such men were inspired by belief in a rational God whose works could be investigated and understood with benefit to mankind.

It is an unfortunate fact, however, that in recent years research in medicine is increasingly being undertaken with inferior motives. The essential object of all clinical study, that of improving the methods which will alleviate suffering and cure disease, is becoming of lesser importance than the quest for knowledge for its own sake or as a means of furthering career prospects. Dr. Szent-Gyorgi, commenting on the character of the research worker, said 'the desire to alleviate suffering is of small value in research – such a person should be advised to work for a charity. Research wants egotists . . . who seek their own pleasure and satisfaction but find it in solving the puzzles of nature'.[6] Although many would take issue with this description applied wholesale to clinical research workers, few doctors would deny that an ingredient of egotism and self satisfaction is present in much modern research work. Moreover self interest tends to be furthered by a system which dictates that a period of full time research work should form a part of training. Publications and theses are produced and added to the curriculum vitae as substantive evidence of endeavour, industry and integrity. Unfortunately many pieces of research performed merely as part of career advancement are embarked upon with undue haste and without sufficient consideration of the need for proper controls, with the inevitable result that no meaningful conclusion can be reached nor can the work be utilized and built upon by other workers in the same field.

There is happily a brighter side to motives in clinical research. Those who stipulate that research should form a part of training do so for good reasons. Research leads to the development of a critical faculty not otherwise readily obtained. An appreciation of the importance of accurate observations and the statistical analysis of results is gained. Not only do these qualities enable objective and honest assessment of one's own work but also encourage perspicacious evaluation of the published results of others. No longer is the printed word accepted as the whole truth solely on the strength of its inclusion in a well known journal or textbook. Instead the research worker is trained to inquire into the foundations upon which published work has been based.

Research on patients makes demands upon the integrity of the doctor and his regard for the personalities of his patients. The high standards of the Christian faith which have helped to lay the foundations of modern medical ethics apply particularly to the field of clinical research where there exists so much potential abuse of the confidence a patient places in his doctor.

### References

1 Ogilvie W. H. Whither Medicine? *Lancet* 1952: 2:820-824.
2 Pappworth M. H. *Human guinea pigs: Experimentation in man.* London: Routledge and Kegan Paul, 1967.
3 Beecher H. K. *Experimentation in man.* Springfield, Illinois: Charles Thomas, 1959.
4 McCance R. A. Practice of experimental medicine. *Proc. R. Soc. Med.* 1951; 44:189-194.
5 Matthew 7:12.
6 Szent-Syorgyi A. Psychiatry: Report on the 3rd World Congress of Psychiatry. *Lancet* 1961; 1:1394.

# 11 Euthanasia
## Duncan Vere

A DEFINITION is essential to any real debate. The term 'euthanasia' has moved from its original usage and has come to mean the deliberate ending of life to relieve suffering. Its chief subdivisions include voluntary euthanasia, requested by the sufferer, which may be fairly described as assisted suicide. This alone has been proposed so far in Britain. Some British proponents, and numbers of American supporters, would go further to compulsory euthanasia – a decision by society to end the life of a sufferer who cannot signify volition. This step is suggested because most of the difficult problems relate to such people as the demented, the deformed infant or the congenital ament.

## Present pressures

Attempts are being made to condition public opinion to accept mercy-killing. Proponents of euthanasia criticize the almost universal emotional distaste for death; euthanasia is called 'giving death' rather than 'taking life'. The withholding of attempts at curative treatments in hopeless cases, long held to be good medical practice, is said to be a form of compulsory euthanasia which doctors practise already. So is the supposedly inevitable respiratory depression which is said to follow increasing morphine dosage in severe pain. Neither assertion is in fact correct. The traditional aims of medicine have been to aid natural recovery, whenever that is likely to be helpful, and always to relieve suffering without deliberately ending life. A doctor who withholds a therapy which is ordinarily curative, because he believes his patient to be incurable, is still assisting nature and leaves recovery an open possibility should his prognosis have been incorrect. For example, to describe the withdrawal of resuscitation when the cerebrum is demonstrably dead as mercy-killing, or as endangering life to relieve suffering, would be akin to arguing that a doctor should never omit any therapy which he thinks to be useless. In severe pain increasing doses of opiates are necessary as their effect dwindles with time. However, it is still possible to obtain relief using increasingly higher doses. The quantity needed to induce respiratory failure increases *pari passu* with that required to relieve pain, though remaining at a higher dose. It is therefore nearly always possible to choose doses which relieve pain without causing death, indeed there is some evidence that those so relieved may even outlive others whose nutrition and rest were disturbed by pain. The exceptions are small numbers of patients who have severe liver or lung disease, or are very young or old and happen to be unusually susceptible to the action of strong analgesics.

Lastly, since much of the opposition to voluntary euthanasia has come from those who believe in a God who cares, their faith has sometimes been attacked on the ground that society needs only their doctrine of mercy without the other doctrines they may preach and practise.

## Is voluntary euthanasia desirable or necessary?

It is most justifiable on the obligation to relieve suffering, and to show mercy. However, it has been repeatedly shown that pain and distress in the period before dying can almost always be effectively relieved given sufficient, but quite ordinary, resources. Where relief is not obtained in our society it is usually because sufficient resources have not been devoted to preterminal care, having been diverted to other more dramatic though worthy health objectives. It is always right to be merciful, but the method need not, and should not, transgress other moral goals.

It is now argued that the Suicide Act of 1962 signified social approval of suicide, and so of assisted suicide. This is not the case. The Act aims only to divert punishment from the unfortunate; severe penalties obtain under the Act for those who assist a suicide.

It is said that increasing numbers of old and infirm people are kept alive by the practice of modern medicine, and that this significantly increases the burdens of over-population. Certainly, if meddlesome medicine is so misapplied as to prolong the act of dying when life is effectively over, that is a great pity. This is not, however, any necessary part of the practice of medicine, nor has it ever been. The population problem has its main roots elsewhere, and is better controlled at the other end of life. Deletion of a few elderly people could not significantly swing its balance, for hardly any of them ask for euthanasia, and those who do wish to die usually prefer to await death naturally.

A strong plea is now advanced for the few intelligent sufferers who wish for voluntary euthanasia on the ground of their individual freedom and their 'right' to choose death, when and as they want it. Unhappily no-one is entirely free, at least from obligations to others, and it is notoriously hard to agree upon human 'rights'. There is at present no agreed 'right' to death. It is likely, as we hope to show below, that the possession of this 'right' would lead to grave infringements of the 'rights' of others, not least other persons' rights to life.

Lastly, it is advanced as a progressive measure that

115

society should freely experiment with every idea which seems practicable, and retain only those which prove satisfactory. It is an unselfish, gentle act to opt out of a useless or degrading life, and so to relieve others of their burden of care. The control of death, like that of life, has now passed on to man. Such notions are not progressive – other communities have tried and rejected them before, though it is often difficult to rid society of unsatisfactory measures once these have become legal. It may not be wise to try to solve dilemmas, which spring from our past decisions about life, by taking greater decisions of a similar kind about death. It is a gentle, generous thing to risk one's life for others, but that is not the same as asking them to take it for oneself. It takes a strong imagination to make the motives of a King Saul coincide with those of a Captain Oates!

There are three strong arguments against voluntary euthanasia: the pressures on patients which would occur, the pressures on doctors and nurses, and the pressures on society. *Patients* could not avoid a sense of unreal obligation to relatives, reading into many incidents at home a spurious (or even real) suggestion that they had better accede to euthanasia. It would be all too easy for the sufferers and their relations to conclude, for different but equally faulty reasons, that their life now held neither point nor purpose.

*Doctors and nurses* would have a changed role in society. Instead of being invariably trusted as acting only to conserve, to relieve and to revive their patients' lives, they would gain a second role. Patients could not be sure where medicine might lead them, and clinical histories and attitudes would be coloured by this fear. The professions would become divided, into those who would and those who would not comply with euthanasia. If, as seems likely, a majority were to refuse there would always be the temptation for the State to turn to others to execute requests, should these eventually exceed the resources of those who were willing to comply.

*The pressures on society.* Inevitably, voluntary would lead to compulsory euthanasia, just as in some places therapeutic abortion has opened the door to abortion on demand. This 'wedge' argument is often derided, but has repeatedly been demonstrated in the enactment. The pressure for compulsory euthanasia would, of course, derive from the large excess of potential candidates for this, as opposed to the voluntary form of euthanasia. Often it is reasonable to suspect the 'wedge' argument as an omnibus reason for inaction. In this context, that would be false complacence; the wedge quickly broadened in Nazi Germany, and mercy might prove an even stronger reason for compulsory euthanasia than utility in some eyes. Suggestions have already been made for delayed euthanasia, using anaesthesia with the guarantee of nonarousal, so that useful experiments could be made on human material. However much the candidate for such euthanasia might have wished his body to be exploited in that way, it could not but cheapen attitudes to human life and over-value human decisions about it.

## Is voluntary euthanasia practicable?

No, because it is impossible to provide adequate safeguards for the patient or for society. Leaving aside the difficulties over insurance, legal status and inheritance, there are three serious problems which override all others. First it must be admitted that the 'I' who signs a paper today is not in all ways the same 'I' who might be deemed to need euthanasia years later, when the paper might be recovered during illness. The real and common problems of a patient's confusion or depression would always make psychiatric assessment mandatory, and impossibly hard to give under such emotional pressures. Medical prognosis is also notoriously uncertain particularly at the time when suffering is at its worst – that is, the preterminal illness when diagnosis may still be uncertain. Lastly, death is a time when families feel guilt, even without euthanasia. What sort of problems would ensue if this guilt were compounded by their consideration, or support of, mercy killing?

## Is voluntary euthanasia right?

Moral decisions are not easy. That there is no self-evident answer in this case is witnessed by the number of clergy who oppose, or propose, euthanasia with transparent integrity. Euthanasia is not murder, which requires a guilty rather than a merciful mind. Nor is the 'sanctity of life' the obvious answer, since it has been upheld by many who took lives freely for other purposes in past centuries. However, all theistic faiths, and most of their adherents, are agreed that life has supreme value, even if not inviolate, and that man is answerable to God for his use of God-given life. The Christian faith upholds the view that man was made like God in some ways (in God's 'image'), that God exerts a providence over life, and that man must answer for his use of it. Mandates are given for life-taking in certain extremes, e.g. the just war or capital punishment. Consideration of the life of Jesus Christ would encourage us to apply healing and mercy without invoking euthanasia. Nowhere is there a mandate given to take innocent life for any reason. Nor is there any place for hopelessness; every sentient person, actual or potential, is seen as having some use and some duty to others. Most Christians would not feel able to share the motives of someone who asked for assisted suicide.

But our society is neither Christian nor theistic. Numbers of people see no moral objection to euthanasia. Is it wrong to deny it to an intelligent, informed person, without relatives or dependents, aged and infirm, suffering from a demonstrable and uniformly fatal malady which will progress steadily through some years of suffering and increasing disablement? Neither he nor his doctor may have any moral objection. Can society insist that they forbear? There is one good reason. Sometimes in ordinary life, as in battle, it seems better for a minority to suffer in order to avert much greater hardship for the whole group. Society has hitherto denied man the 'right' to assisted suicide in order to conserve wider freedoms. It is so easy to struggle to secure the rights and privileges of an esoteric few only to discover that the many suffer disproportionately in the process.

Because euthanasia runs counter to a positive view of human life, because it would apply pressure to the healing professions to do something foreign to their calling and debase their social function, and because it would risk compulsory euthanasia, it seems better to avoid it altogether. There are other means to relieve suffering. There is no need to change the law, either to provide voluntary euthanasia or to divert resources from other spheres where they are urgently required, in order to bring the appropriate care to the dying and those with chronic, severe disabilities. Our society certainly should not shirk its burden of caring for these suffererers by taking steps to eliminate those in need – even should they request this for themselves. Their plea is magnanimous, but mistaken.

## A positive alternative

It is arguable that voluntary euthanasia, however distasteful it may be, is the lesser evil – less objectionable than protracted suffering or despair. This argument accepts evils as they are. We may attempt to change them. It is said that the law requires reform. Why not aim to reform society instead? Suffering in chronic illness is only partly due to the disease. It is when we 'save life', without alleviating pain or disability, that it is at its worst. Good preterminal care brings the sufferer back out of painful isolation to be a member of society again. Pain is not an absolute. Like all sensations it is subject to competition. Several specialized hospitals for the dying have shown what can be achieved. The principles so learned have been barely applied in the

National Health Service so far. This is because good care is costly, chiefly in terms of human effort and devotion. Too few are motivated to help care for dying persons in our society, and their work is economically unproductive and unexciting. It is cheaper and easier to take people's lives to end their sufferings. Sadly, it is also true that much failure to relieve pain springs from ignorance of the pharmacology of opiates, despite the fact that those are among the oldest remedies in general use. The facts are not simple, but they can be learned with a modicum of effort.[1]

Ultimately we must decide whether social structures are organized for the sake of the people who constitute them or whether people exist for society or what is a just balance between these two extremes. If some people want euthanasia we must decide whether to grant them that 'liberty' or whether to improve society so that they no longer want it. By a curious paradox, the best for the individual is not found by considering him in isolation from his society, even if it be agreed that his society should exist to meet his needs. Our argument is that euthanasia, practised for the individual's 'benefit', would cause his society so to deteriorate as to cement its harshness into permanence, and so hurt both him and others. It is therefore better, if costlier, to change the attitude of society so that it supports the individual sufferer in his illness and so that care ousts despair and a person's worth expressed becomes a worth experienced.

### References

[1] Twycross R. G. Relief of terminal pain. *Br. Med. J.* 1975; 4:212-214.

### Further Reading

Brand P. W. *Is life really sacred?* London: CMF Publications, 1973.

Twycross R. G. *The dying patient.* London: CMF Publications, 1975.

Vere D. W. *Voluntary Euthanasia – is there an alternative?* 2nd Ed. London: CMF Publications, 1979.

Searle J. F. *Kill or Care?* Exeter: Paternoster Press, 1977.

## 12   Dilemmas in paediatrics

John Tripp

DOCTORS concerned with the investigation and treatment of children are faced with certain moral and ethical dilemmas which are peculiar to this particular field. As in other branches of medicine the physician's first duty is to the patient, although in paediatric practice the wishes and best interest of the child or infant may be difficult or impossible to ascertain, since as fully dependent members of a family, their parents must actually take the decisions for them. That the physician's primary responsibility is to the child is emphasized in the recent Children's Act (1976)[1] where provision is made for the child to be formally represented at care proceedings by a person other than the parents (or their representative) or the representative of the Social Services Department. Routine clinical decisions and occasionally those affecting the survival of the child have often, however, to be taken in the light of family circumstances and therefore conflicts of interest and moral dilemmas may arise. More often than not, however, the interests of the child and family coincide even in the most difficult areas of decision-making.

An adult with advanced cancer given a ten per cent chance of complete success might reasonably refuse an operation but who is to make such a decision for an infant or child? The newborn infant with a major congenital malformation is an example of the kind of ethical dilemma faced by paediatricians.

## Congenital malformations

A paediatric surgeon[2] has suggested that infants born with severe malformations can be classified into four groups, and his arrangement can be modified to include biochemical disorders:

1. Infants with abnormalities which are incompatible with life if untreated, but where established methods of treatment result in complete recovery and the expectation of normal life. Such conditions as oesophageal atresia and phenylketonuria come in this category.

2. Infants with severe disorders, which are incompatible with life even with present day treatment. Under this heading might be included anencephaly and certain of the neurolipidoses, e.g. Niemann-Pick disease, infantile Gaucher's disease.

3. Infants with a correctable condition in association with an underlying or separate condition, which although not immediately fatal, will mean that the child will never lead an entirely normal life. Examples are a mongol child with jejunal atresia or a child with cystic fibrosis with meconium ileus and neonatal pneumonia.

4. Infants with severe abnormalities which are likely, but by no means certain, to be fatal without intervention, but are only partially correctable, and may in association with other defects mean that the surviving child has severe mental and/or physical handicaps. An example of such a situation is the infant born with an open myelomeningocoele complicated by hydrocephalus, paraplegia or other major disorder.

The clinical, ethical and moral decisions to be taken

when the infant has a disorder which can be classified in groups 1 or 2 is not difficult. In group 3 treatment should be active partly because of the difficulties of making an accurate prognosis regarding future development at the time when the decision has to be taken, which is usually in the first few days of life. A child who is in the fourth category, however, presents a dilemma as there are ethical problems whichever course is chosen.

The example of the infant with a myelomeningocoele is a useful model, as much is known about the prognosis with, and without, treatment. As surgical techniques for repair of such defects advanced, it became common for surgeons to offer surgery to all patients and preserve life by any means possible. Some of the infants who were 'saved' in the neonatal period lived only a few years, during which time they were continually in and out of hospital for reconstructive surgery, urinary diversion, shunting of CSF for hydrocephalus, orthopaedic manoeuvres to help paraplegia, and the many complications of frequent operations. Such surgical feats in the neonatal period combined with good medical care may save a life for a few years and be described as 'heroic'. In reality, the heroism is required of the child and his family not of the surgeon, paediatrician or nursing staff. It is only comparatively recently that it has been suggested that some selection should take place using sound clinical criteria. Operations are now generally performed only when the results are likely to be favourable in the long term. It has been proposed[3] that infants who have not been selected for active surgical management should be given only routine nursing care with attention to relief of pain and suffering and not subjected to therapeutic manoeuvres. Only a very few such infants survive to reach their first birthday, most dying within the first months of life and there is no evidence in this group that withholding early surgery results in any increase in their already severe handicaps.

The medical staff may have the unpleasant and demanding task of telling the parents the truth about the future and the fact that operation, although prolonging life, will not 'cure' the new baby and may result in the prolongation of a miserable existence. If, on the other hand, the parents are told that 'We will do all we can,' it may become impossible to decide, morally and emotionally, when to stop treatment. Suffering may thereby be inflicted on the child, and enormous strains placed on the family. In this situation marital relations are often stressed to the uttermost. Parents find their responsibilities to each other and their normal children very difficult to combine with care for the severely handicapped child. The sequelae of this situation may be the maladjustment of children or severe marital problems.

The fact that there is much useful information about the quality of physical and mental life in a given neonatal situation helps considerably in making rational decisions in these circumstances. Recent surveys of opinion among paediatricians and surgeons in the USA[4,5] suggest that there is broad general agreement as to which infants should not be offered surgery although most leave the final decision to parents after adequate explanation of the likely outcome and prognosis.

In some ways decisions in this situation are easier than those which have to be taken regarding the prolonged use of life support systems in children who have, for example, severe brain damage as a result of injury or illness in later childhood.

## Christian principles

This problem has so far been discussed in purely practical terms. We have examined the possible results of a decision to treat, or not to treat, without taking moral standards into account. The Christian doctor's approach will be based on an understanding of the principles taught by Christ which are often amplified and explained in other parts of the Bible. The Christian believes that life itself is God given and maintained both in the creation of the organism (the body) and more importantly in the life which God 'breathed into man', setting him apart from the rest of creation. That our life is God's to give or take away has led some to suggest that the practice of medicine is wrong for a Christian, as it shows a lack of faith in God's promises. However, the fact that Luke was a practising physician and Jesus gave His disciples authority to heal are surely evidence that we should use our God-given knowledge and skills in the practice of medicine.

We need to realize, nevertheless, that our medical knowledge can be applied inappropriately. It seems unlikely that God ever intended us to use the art of healing to create suffering, as is possible in the circumstances already discussed. Perhaps the most relevant statement in support of this argument are the words of Christ's commandment 'Love your neighbour as yourself.' Can we in all honesty say that we are loving our patients and their families if by saving a life we merely create the kind of problems previously described? It has been argued that by failing to use the skills we have to keep an infant alive, we are in fact aiding his death and are therefore guilty of breaking the 6th commandment. In fact, we are merely allowing natural processes to take their course, because we know that to prolong life in this situation would be to increase suffering.

## Children with handicaps

Having dealt with this difficult situation at some length, it is important to emphasize that it is only comparatively rarely that this situation is met, since the majority of children born with congenital abnormalities fall into one of the other categories in our original classification. Nevertheless some patients will grow up with varying degrees of mental and physical handicaps and in caring for these families there is a real challenge to be met.

Our primary aim is to improve the wellbeing and happiness of the child in a family setting. Lorber[2] has summarized it succinctly as being 'to add life to their years rather than years to their lives'.

A Christian doctor should be the last person (but often is not) to fall into the trap of treating the physical and psychological needs of the child, while ignoring the tremendous problems which may arise in the family unit because to deal with them takes understanding, time and immense patience and is emotionally upsetting for both doctor and family. Only by showing real concern for every detail of the child's care – including the mobilization of local authority services and financial help – and giving sufficient time for the anxious parents to dissipate some of their problems on the already overworked doctor, can we begin to fulfil our Lord's command. Our compassion should be evident to the parents so that they are able to unburden themselves and, perhaps, in our attitude see something of the caring of Christ himself. Only a real personal understanding between parent and doctor will allow sufficient interchange of ideas for the parents to take full advantage of the support of our welfare state and give their child the best care. This may be especially important if it becomes necessary for the child to go into long term care, when the parents need implicit trust in their medical advisers.

As Christian doctors our responsibility is to relieve suffering. In achieving this end we may have to make difficult clinical, moral and ethical decisions. Our aim must be to show to our patients that the love that Christ has taught us is all-embracing and enables us to give of ourselves in helping those in our care.

## Paediatric research

The principle of informed consent is a basic tenet in all codes of conduct used for the examination and control of research methods and protocols. There is ample freedom for the research worker in this situation, since patients are normally willing to participate fully in properly run and controlled research programmes. When considering research in children, however, the situation becomes considerably more complex. Fully informed consent is usually impossible to obtain from children (and obviously so from infants). Furthermore, there is doubt as to whether a parent is legally qualified to give consent for any procedure that is not of direct benefit to the child. Taking the legal aspect first, it has been stated that the law does not allow any investigation or procedure to be carried out on a child (whether it be a blood pressure measurement or a liver biopsy) that is not of direct benefit to the child. To date this position has never been fully tested in the courts of this country.

In fact this rigid legal position is far from secure and doubt has been cast on it, notably by Skegg[9], who suggests that many children may give legal consent, and that a parent may give consent for their child in a situation where a 'reasonable parent'[10] might give consent. Dworkin[11] and others[12] also conclude that research in children is both legal and ethical and suggest guidelines similar to those indicated below.

In practice, paediatric research trials are so designed that:

(a) only procedures of negligible risk are undertaken,

(b) strict monitoring of research projects allows only those projects which are likely to be helpful and have not previously been undertaken. In addition the trials are arranged so as to minimize interference with the patient. For example, a blood sample for 'research' is taken at the same time as blood is taken for therapeutic reasons.

(c) the purpose and nature of the research is fully explained to the parents (and child, if old enough) and their consent obtained.

Public concern over investigative procedures, both in

minors and adults, centres on the protection of the rights and freedom of the individual. In children where these rights are not legally satisfied by informed consent, research immediately becomes out of bounds. On the other hand without paediatric research we should not have been able to achieve the enormous reduction in childhood mortality and morbidity that has occurred;[13] there seems little doubt that the practice of research in children is beneficial to society as a whole. Thus there are two conflicting responsibilities: one to the individual and the other to the society in which we live. While it is simple enough to advocate a ban on paediatric research this would mean that no benefits would accrue to society, which might be as unjustifiable as causing a child pain.

Why have rights and freedom of the individual assumed such importance in our society – as compared to many others where individual rights are always secondary to those of the community? The answer almost certainly is the strong emphasis on the infinite worth of the individual in Christian teaching, particularly in the New Testament, which has been fundamental in the foundation of our legal and social codes. The extreme disregard for individual freedom in the name of the community and medicine by the Nazis resulted in several declarations of medical ethics,[14] all of which sought to redress the balance in favour of the individual. It has been suggested[15] that this has resulted in over-compensation, so that now it is the rights of the community that have been neglected. Examination of both Old and New Testaments certainly suggests that while we have a responsibility to God, we also have a responsibility to our fellows and society as a whole. This must surely lend weight to the possibility that carefully controlled research in children may be both justifiable and desirable.[16]

In conclusion, those involved in paediatric research must take the utmost care in clinical trial design to ensure that the research is essential, organized so as to give a minimal risk-to-benefit ratio and is undertaken only with the fullest possible consent of parent and child.

## References

1. Eckstein H. B. Severely malformed children. *Br. Med. J.* 1973; 2:284.
2. Lorber J. Ethical problems in the management of myelomeningocoele and hydrocephalus. *J. R. Coll. Physicians, London* 1975; 10:47-59.
3. Shaw A. *et. al.* Ethical issues in pediatric surgery. *Pediatrics* 1977; 60:588-599.
4. Todres I. D. *et. al.* Pediatricians attitudes affecting decision-making in defective newborns. *Pediatrics* 1977; 60:197-201.
5. MacLachlan G. *Patient, doctor and society.* London: Oxford University Press, 1972.
6. Genesis 2:7.
7. Job 12:10.
8. James 4:14-16.
9. Skegg P. D. G. English Law relating to experimentation on children. *Lancet* 1977; 2:754-755.
10. S.V. McC., W. v. W., 1972. AC24 (House of Lords).
11. Dworkin G. Legality of consent to non-therapeutic medical research on infants and young children. *Arch Dis Child* 1978; 53:443-446.
12. Editorial. Research on children. *Br. Med. J.* 1978; 2:1043-1044.
13. Lowe C. U., Alexander D., Mishkin B. Nontherapeutic research on children: An ethical dilemma. *J. Pediat.* 1974; 84:468-472.
14. The Nuremberg Code, the Helsinki Declaration and the statement by the British Medical Research Council.
15. Porter A. M. W. Research investigations in children. *Br. Med. J.* 1973; 2:403.
16. Suran B. G., Lavigne J. V. Rights of children in pediatric settings. *Pediatrics* 1977; 60:715-720.

## Further Reading

Ethics of selective treatment of spina bifida: Report by a working party. *Lancet* 1975; 1:85-88.

Johnsen A. R. Research involving children. Recommendations of the National Committee for the protection of human subjects of bio-medical and behavioural research. *Pediatrics* 1978; 62:131-136.

## 13  Unwanted pregnancy

Christine Tuck

AMONG the patients attending most gynaecological clinics in this country will be some requesting abortion. 'The next patient wants a termination,' says the nurse, and the doctor is faced by one of the more acute ethical problems of modern medical practice. Yet, in fact, the doctor is being consulted by an anxious patient who needs help with a problem which is usually very distressing to her – an unwanted pregnancy. Some will be young unmarried girls wearing the latest fashion, with beautiful shining hair streaming over their shoulders. Others will be mothers of large impoverished families, old beyond their years; the accompanying children may disturb their concentration. Some come with tales of desertion, fears of malformed babies, or the prospect of a shattered professional career. Some are distraught; some angry; some insolent; some depressed and withdrawn. They each need help, understanding and compassion. It is in this context that we must consider whether their pregnancy should be terminated.

With the rest of the Profession, Christian doctors inevitably meet this problem, whether or not they are gynaecologists. Their attitudes need to be soundly based and clear, so that Christ is honoured in this, as in every other, aspect of their lives.   As St. Paul said, 'Let your conduct be worthy of the gospel of Christ. . . .'[1]

## Facts

The 1967 Abortion Act came into force in April 1968, permitting abortion when it is considered that (a) the continuance of the pregnancy would involve risk to the life of the pregnant woman, or of injury to the physical or mental health of the woman or any existing children of her family, greater than if the pregnancy were terminated; or (b) that there is a substantial risk that, if the child were born, it would suffer from such physical or mental abnormalities as to be seriously handicapped. Two doctors have to agree in good faith that one or more of these conditions apply.   Also, the operation has to be conducted in an approved hospital or nursing home.   The Act includes a clause permitting people with conscientious objections to opt out of the working of the Act.

Each year in England and Wales one fetus is legally aborted for every six babies born alive.   In 1978, 112,055 legal abortions were performed on residents. This means that about 1 per cent of all women of child-bearing age had an abortion in that year; over 3,000 of these operations were on children under 16 years of age. Nearly 80 per cent of all the operations were done to protect the physical or mental health of the mother (Clause II, Abortion Act).

As with any other operation complications may occur. The incidence of death, sepsis, haemorrhage or acute psychosis is fairly easily assessed, but the resultant incidence of secondary infertility can only be roughly estimated.   (Suggested figures range from 3-28 per cent.) However, it is extremely difficult to produce even a rough estimate for other long term effects of abortion, which may be equally damaging, such as the regrets of the mother who has had a termination, the morbid fear of many women that a subsequent baby will be abnormal as a 'punishment', or the effect that the knowledge that their mother has had a termination may have on the other children in the family.

Requests for termination in the general practitioners' surgeries and in the hospital clinics increase. Techniques improve; but the inevitable and sad sequelae also continue to become apparent.

## Guidelines

Christians have had to give urgent consideration to the ethical and moral questions raised by abortion.

The termination of a pregnancy cannot be considered in the same way as, for instance, the prophylactic appendicectomy required of intending polar explorers. The fetus is not merely an inessential organ of the mother to be removed as a matter of convenience. It is a potential independent human person. Biblical teaching is clear that individual human life is precious in the sight of God because man is made in His image[2] and through the sacrifice of Jesus Christ man is offered the sonship of God.[3] Therefore the status of the fetus has to be carefully considered.

In Jeremiah[4] we read, 'Before I formed you in the womb, I knew you, and before you were born I consecrated you,' showing God's caring concern for the unborn. However, Rex Gardner, a Christian gynaecologist, suggests[5] that, in the light of some modern research, it may be wrong to presume that human life is sacred from the moment of fertilization. He mentions that in some forms of twinning, division of the embryo does not occur until after implantation; hence, it must be asked 'Does the soul also split?' He cites the problem of regarding a morula developed from an *in vitro* fertilization as a human. He also discusses the problems inherent in regarding all early spontaneous abortions (possibly 50 per cent of all conceptions) as lost human lives. For this would mean that the greater proportion of humans would never reach fetal maturity.

Blunt[6] has suggested that we should be concerned to discover the time at which a fetus becomes a person. He relates personality to an ability to respond to fellow human beings and this to an ability to respond to God. The crucial stage in the development of the fetus would therefore depend on a minimal development of the nervous system, without which such response is impossible. Many commentators suggest that, in Exodus 21: 22,23, maternal life is considered more precious than fetal life because the penalty for inflicting maternal injury is more severe than the fine imposed for inducing abortion. However, despite these ideas many would agree with Dietrich Bonhoeffer when he wrote 'To raise the question whether we are here concerned with a human being, or not, is merely to confuse the issue. The simple fact is that God certainly intended to create a human being, and that this nascent human being has been deliberately deprived of his life. And this is nothing short of murder.'[7] It should, however, be noted that in law and legal phraseology, the use of the word 'murder' implies the concept of 'malice aforethought' associated with the act of killing. A better term in this translation would be 'manslaughter'.

Is every abortion, therefore, a form of homicide? This is not merely a theoretical question, but of practical importance especially to the Christian patient seeking a termination, or a doctor about to perform one. The sixth commandment,[8] 'You shall not kill' is often quoted to show that Christians should have nothing to do with abortions. But the meaning of the verb as 'illegal killing inimical to the community' needs to be weighed, and in this light not all abortions induced in this country can be considered homicide however the phrase 'inimical to the community' is interpreted.

## Practical considerations

If abortion is justified in some circumstances, these need to be clearly defined. Some Christians have no difficulty in accepting Clause I of the 1967 Abortion Act, under which an abortion may be procured if the continuance of the pregnancy threatens the life of the mother. This, however, is an exceptional situation, and represents only 0.5 per cent of all abortions performed in 1978. About 89 per cent were performed under clauses II and III (risk to the mother's or children's mental or physical health). It is in this group that there is likely to be most divergence of opinion. As an American has put it: in order to get an abortion 'many women gladly have themselves declared psychiatrically unstable'.[9]

Some writers have tried to draw a distinction between the physical and mental health of the mother and her social situation; but probably the whole picture should be taken together and the foreseeable social situation included. This necessarily includes the children of the family. It is this clause which, liberally interpreted, allows abortion on demand, because overall maternal mortality statistics (without regard to age and parity of the patient) suggests that she is less likely to die if she has an abortion, than if she continues with the pregnancy. The Christian is unlikely to agree with this interpretation in that it completely negates the right of the fetus. However, it can be difficult to counter the taunt, usually from humanists, that, in trying to make a reasoned decision for each individual patient, one is playing judge and failing to be consistently loving. Yet, the unwanted pregnancy is often merely a symptom of many complex underlying problems, such as alcoholism, and it is, therefore, facile to assume that abortion is necessarily even a part of the best management of the whole situation. The taunt also betrays a very superficial understanding of 'love' by New Testament standards.

In trying to help such a patient an attempt has to be made to achieve the right decision from all possible view points, though these may ultimately prove irreconcilable. The decision must be right from the patient's point of view, with due regard to her total situation in so far as she is willing to share it. Most obstetricians have from time to time delivered a child for a patient who has ultimately been grateful that her original request for termination was refused. The discovery of an unexpected pregnancy, perhaps especially when contraceptive precuations fail, can lead to panic and despair at a time when the patient is least able to view matters rationally. The crisis often comes when she is most affected by the disturbing physiological changes associated with pregnancy. In some patients a plea for termination is merely a plea for support in recognizing and adjusting to a pregnancy. It may also prove an unspoken request for support against the impulsive reaction of a husband overwhelmed by the prospect of another child in the family.

This decision must also be in accord with the doctor's conscience and be regarded in a positive context. It may be that a decision for abortion is made as the lesser of two evils, but it must be made confidently because the patient may need the reassurance of such confidence in adjusting to the final decision. So for most Christians, a decision concerning abortion is often difficult. It cannot be used, as so many would wish it to be, as a cheap substitute for the patient herself in the burdensome responsibility of motherhood, or for society in the provision of adequate housing and social services. A potential human life is at stake. If all patients were Christian then many of the problems, faced by doctors concerned with abortion, would be much reduced. But, in our imperfect world, it is our first duty to serve our Lord and, in the light of that, our privilege to serve our patients humbly.

Clause IV of the Abortion Act allows the termination of pregnancy where there is a substantial risk that the child would be seriously handicapped. How can the adjectives 'substantial' and 'seriously' be assessed in this context? Can it be right to abort all pregnancies where the first four weeks have been complicated by maternal rubella because there would be a 47 per cent risk of fetal abnormality? Clearly, over half the fetuses aborted would be normal. And it must be reckoned that some people who have lived joyful lives and been a blessing to their family can only be categorized as 'severely handicapped'. Techniques of antenatal diagnosis allow us to quantify 'substantial' in some cases. For instance chromosome analysis of the cells in the liquor amnii can give a definite diagnosis of mongolism. However, other tests, such as $\alpha$-fetoprotein levels for detecting open neural tube defects, give results which are much more difficult to interpret, have a recognized false positive rate, do not give 100 per cent pick-up, and indicate only a very broad spectrum of abnormality.[10] Also, the methods involved in achieving an antenatal diagnosis of fetal abnormality may involve a greater risk to the fetus than the risk of a detectable abnormality being present.[11] (E.g. Amniocentesis carries a risk of causing abortion of about 1.5 per cent. The risk of a 35-year-old woman having a mongol child is only about 0.9 per cent). Thus accurate and detailed information is necessary to evaluate the possible benefits and dangers for the individual patient. The scope of antenatal diagnosis is extending and will allow an increasing number of parents to know that their baby would be handicapped in a particular way, although not necessarily the severity of the handicap. The parental anxiety engendered may be overwhelming as these investigations proceed, and painstaking explanations are required at all stages. As screening tests on maternal blood are increasingly employed, this need for sympathetic communication will similarly increase as doubtful results and repeat tests play havoc with the mother's peace of mind. Christian doctors have to decide whether the presence of a particular abnormality should be grounds for a termination of pregnancy; almost always the total context of the pregnancy must be taken into account as with any other reason for abortion.

## Conclusion

Among Christian doctors opinions differ as to the right attitude to abortion, from those who believe that such a procedure should never be entertained to those who regard the termination of an unwanted pregnancy as merely a logical extension of a responsible family planning programme. We need to listen to each other and respect each other's views, but we all need to recognize that unwanted pregnancies frequently occur because of poor family relationships, loneliness or ignorance. Often, in retrospect, it is easy to identify the women at risk. Loving and sometimes sacrificial efforts are needed to change these people and their circumstances before the tragedy of an unwanted pregnancy occurs and the request for a termination is made. However, if it is accepted that termination of pregnancy may be the right response to some requests, the best possible conditions in which to discuss the decision and sufficient time must be made available for each patient, so that her problems can be carefully considered and all possible avenues explored in achieving a decision about which both patient and doctor can be at peace. For instance, a brief telephone conversation with the general practitioner or a home visit by a social worker may transform one's appreciation of the problems. The patient with the greatest burdens is often the least articulate or demanding.[12] Arrangements must also be made so that the views of one's colleagues, who do not agree with termination on any account, can be respected. For instance, abortions can always be put in the same section of an operating list.

Termination of pregnancy can never be lightly entered into, but in performing such an operation a Christian can find fulfilment in the knowledge that he is continuing his walk with our Lord and Saviour Jesus Christ. For as we read in Micah, 'He has showed you, O man, what is good; and what does the Lord require of you but to do justice, and to love kindness, and to walk humbly with your God?'[13] Feelings are dangerous, but the 'natural' revulsion most surgeons, Christian and otherwise, feel during a termination, as a potential human life is destroyed, will always remind us of the enormous responsibility we have accepted in reaching our decision. It is only by prayerfully following the guiding principles we have been given that we can hope to be faithful to our duty to be 'the salt of the earth'[14] in this difficult area.

### References

[1] Philippians 1:27.
[2] Genesis 1:27.
[3] Romans 8:15-17.
[4] Jeremiah 1:5.
[5] Gardner, R. F. R. *Abortion – the personal dilemma.* Exeter: The Paternoster Press, 1972.
[6] Blunt M. Human life and the human person. *Interchange* 1968; 1:No. 4.
[7] Bonhoeffer D. *Ethics.* London: Fontana, 1963.
[8] Exodus 20:13.
[9] Henry C. F. H. *Facing the abortion crisis. J. Christian Med. Soc.* 1971.
[10] Stirrat G. M. *et. al.* Clinical dilemmas arising from the antenatal diagnosis of neural tube defects. *Br. J. Obstet. Gynaecol.* 1979; 86:161-166.
[11] An assessment of the hazards of amniocentesis. *Br. J. Obstet. Gynaecol.* 1978; 85:Supp. 2.
[12] Dunlop J. L. Counselling of patients requesting an abortion. *Practitioner* 1978; 220:847-852.
[13] Micah 6:8.
[41] Matthew 5:13.

### Further Reading

Stirrat G. M. *Legalised abortion.* London: CMF Publications, 1979.

# 14  Geriatric medicine

George Chalmers

It is becoming increasingly difficult to be engaged in the clinical practice of medicine without being involved in the care of the aged. One might escape by becoming a paediatrician, or perhaps an obstetrician, but the latter's involvement with gynaecology would re-assert the reality of the 'ageing population'. The general physician, the general surgeon, the general practitioner, the psychiatrist, neurologist, haematologist and endocrinologist – indeed every doctor concerned in the medical care of adult people – is becoming progressively aware of the rise in the average age of the patients who make demands upon time and attention in hospital and in the community. Thirteen per cent of the population of the United Kingdom is of pensionable age, and between now and the turn of the century there will be a thirty-five per cent increase in the number of people over 75 years of age in the community.

It is as a result of this population growth in the upper age groups that the specialty of geriatric medicine has come into being. It may well be concluded that, increasingly, the medicine of the elderly is the general medicine of the eighties, particularly as the field of the traditional general physician becomes more and more specialized.

**The nature of geriatrics**

For this reason it is difficult to define the specialty in precise terms, and it has been suggested that the basic difference between the geriatric physician and the general physician lies in the realm of attitudes rather than activities. Unhappily one still meets colleagues whose negative attitudes towards the elderly in their practice do them no honour as physicians. We are neither concerned, nor content, to provide a mere custodial or caretaker type of care for old people, who require to be 'looked after' with the minimum of 'disturbance' in the way of investigation or even treatment until they may be 'left alone to die in peace'. The fallacy of such an attitude lies in the tragedy of undiagnosed, remediable disease, and the demonstrable fact that, if the elderly are 'left alone', they very often die in neither peace nor comfort. Diagnostic and therapeutic nihilism have no place in the practice of any kind of medicine, and least of all in geriatric medicine. The medical management of the elderly patient demands the same diagnostic acumen, the same critical use of the technology of medicine, and the same involved, practical compassion as one should find in good medical care at any age. Specific to the field is the emphasis on rehabilitation based on the study of disability, and on the co-ordination of services in the community to meet the needs of the elderly in terms of the prevention of disease, and its treatment, management and support. Geriatrics has been defined recently as 'the strenuous art of exhausting the possible on the patient's behalf' and it is only when one is prepared to discard the attitude that 'nothing can be done' that one begins to learn just how much is included in 'the possible'.

The patient reputedly suffering from 'senility', on examination, turns out to have not only a multiple pathology whose nature can be clearly defined element by element but also a surprisingly remediable content within that pathology. The disparaging term 'senile', can cover undiagnosed myxoedema, pernicious anaemia, scurvy, subdural haematoma and a number of other conditions which respond just as well to treatment at 75 as they do at 45. The hazards of the diagnostic 'ragbag' of the 'degenerative diseases' may well be blinding us to the potential for recovery which might be realized following adequate assessment and investigation. This will demand discernment, effort and well informed discipline, as well as the compassion, kindness and sympathy which are integral to the management of the elderly and the disabled. No-one need fear professional or intellectual stagnation in the practice of the medicine of old age.

## The importance of motivation

To the Christian in particular the challenge in medicine is to care, to be touched, as the Lord himself was, with the feeling of our infirmities and with those of our fellow men. Nowhere is there more opportunity in our present society than in the geriatric realm, for so very often the poor, the widowed, the halt, the lame, the blind and the lonely are to be found predominantly among the elderly, despite the financial and other provisions made by the welfare state. There is still human need in our society, which lays a claim upon informed, trained compassion, and which constitutes a challenge to care.

Disease in the later years of life is often less dramatic than in the younger person. Its elucidation is not only a clamant necessity for the sufferer, who, not recognizing it as disease, may be blaming the inevitability of old age for his disability, but is equally a stimulating study in the interaction of the personality, the environment and the physical limitations of the individual. One of the fascinations to me personally in practice among elderly people has been to see vignettes of the kind of people the Lord healed in His earthly ministry. The man by the pool of Siloam, who had so given up hope that he could only answer with a complaint, when the Lord asked 'Do you want to recover?'[1] The persistent, demanding, unremitting claim of Bartimaeus who will not be put off.[2] The touching reticence of the woman who had suffered from haemorrhages for twelve years who didn't want to be a bother, but would be satisfied with the touch of the hem of His garment[3] – believing that she might thereby be healed. They are all there, and although our diagnostic and therapeutic skills are so limited in comparison to the Saviour's, we may still give, in His Name, of the fruits of our study and expertise in our various fields to those who may be 'the least of all these, My brethren'.[4]

We have a responsibility to avoid a double standard of care; a situation in which the 'interesting' (i.e. the relatively rare or dramatic presentation of illness with a 'satisfying' management or outcome) receives the larger part of our attention, and the 'ordinary' or the 'chronic' a much lesser share. Stroke illness is an excellent example of this distinction, and one in which the assumption that 'all strokes are the same' is readily refuted by adequate examination and investigation. The left-sided stroke with perceptive loss, neglect, denial of disease, and even mis-identification of the limb as belonging to someone else. The variations of communications disorder in the dysphasia of the right-sided stroke patient. The effects of brain damage in each situation. The interplay of intercurrent and co-incidental illness. The response of physical rehabilitation to the treatment of depression. There is no end to the fascination of this 'dull and routine' type of illness. When the stroke patient is given the 'interesting case' kind of clinical attention and is the focus of attention of a diagnostic and therapeutic rehabilitative team, the result in terms of function may be surprising – and, even if it is not, we have still the responsibility to go on trying and to go on caring.

Long-term illness is exacting in its demands upon the doctor, as upon nursing and other staff. The maintenance of interest in someone whose condition varies little from week to week and from month to month can prove extremely difficult, if one is inclined to think in terms of clinical interest only. In this situation it is necessary to look beyond the pathology to the person, and the question of relationship becomes paramount. Old age is a time of failing relationship, in which so many on whom the person has come to depend are, for one reason or another, withdrawn or no longer available. In this situation it is a great deal more than a platitude to suggest that the relationship forged between the doctor and the elderly person may be at least as effective as any medication prescribed by him.

For the Christian doctor the outworking of the 'hope that is in us'[5] may well make that relationship therapeutic in a spiritual as well as in a physical, social or psychological sense. If the faith which distinguishes us as Christians is real, it will have an effect upon our lives, and it will affect our professional life no less than our private life. Old people do consider such issues, and the opportunity to 'give a reason' for that hope is not as rare as might be imagined. The slower turnover, the longer hospital stay, the slower pace of activity in a continuing care geriatric ward will often mean that the doctor, from resident to consultant, is seen more readily as a person. It is with people, rather than with 'busy doctors', that the people who are patients will talk about such matters.

## Professional satisfaction

In terms of professional satisfaction this field of medicine is as full and as rewarding as any other, provided the temperament of the doctor is compatible with the demands of this exacting discipline.

In terms of professional advancement the opportunities are better than in the general medical and surgical fields, and research opportunity is wide, but as a motivation these alone may well prove insufficient.

In terms of opportunity for service for the Christian in medicine, I believe the medicine of old age is unparalleled. It is a field in which Christian compassion, concern and involvement can add a major dimension to the care of people whose needs are multiple and compounded of physical, psychological, social and spiritual elements.

**References**

[1] John 5:6.
[2] Mark 10:48.
[3] Matthew 9:20.
[4] Matthew 25:40.
[5] 1 Peter 3:15.

## 15  Psychiatry
### Montagu Barker

MANY medical students find psychiatry a disturbing subject within the curriculum. Sometimes Christian students find it particularly so. The purpose of this chapter is to explore some of the reasons for this.

### New concepts

Hitherto our training and concepts of illness have been based upon the natural sciences. Our teachers have spoken with a fair degree of unanimity and authority. We have learned to diagnose illness by such means as sight and touch, backed up by a plethora of sophisticated laboratory tests. We have learned to treat illness with drugs specific to the particular condition, or by means of an operation for the removal of diseased tissue.

In psychiatry much of the teaching is based upon the new behavioural sciences. Aetiology is now discussed frequently in terms of the effect of his environment upon the patient, and the difficulties he may have in interpersonal relationships. The clinical features noted are disordered behaviour, anomalies of mood and disturbed thinking and perception. Physical methods of treatment are used; but treatment frequently consists of psychotherapy, the verbal interchange between therapist and patient, which to some may seem to be mere chat. Another new factor is that there seem to be so many schools of thought among psychiatrists, ranging from those who take an organic approach to mental illness to those who take a Freudian psychoanalytical approach, while others unashamedly combine both extremes.

This new understanding of illness, its causes and treatment, coupled with the lack of unanimity among his teachers, may create in the student a feeling of unease. This may result in his rejecting the subject completely.

## Personal involvement

Previously, in our study of medicine, we have progressed from the study of matter and the basic sciences to the study of lower forms of life, which was followed by the study of the human body, and finally the study of diseased function in the living body. This materialistic approach to illness has always been combined in the good physician with a real concern for the patient as a person. However, when dealing with physical illnesses it is much easier to ignore the person who is ill and concentrate upon his lesions and pathology.

In dealing with a patient who is mentally ill this detachment is much more difficult. This is partly because psychiatric case history-taking is much more detailed than the case history-taking with which we have been familiar so far. For instance we have to record the patient's reaction to his parents, his marital relationships, his response to crisis and stress, and his feelings and attitudes towards a wide variety of situations. Inevitably, as we look more closely at how the patient deals with life and those around him, we ourselves become involved and compare our own attitudes with his. We certainly react in some way. We may sympathize with the patient so much that we become unduly involved, or we may find ourselves becoming critical and so reject the patient.

In addition to this, as we learn about the way in which

the mind works, we gain insight into the way in which we habitually cope with stress in our own lives. For some this is disturbing. Also, as we hear about the nature of psychiatric symptoms, we should not be medical students if we did not introspect a little and do a symptom inventory upon ourselves. The discovery of similarities between ourselves and our patients does not of course indicate illness any more than a pain in the chest indicates a heart attack. However the fear that we share some of the symptoms of our patients may cause us to protect ourselves – either by rejecting psychiatry and those who suffer from mental illness, or by becoming over-involved with our patients, hoping thereby to solve our own problems. This is why in psychiatry part of the training is directed towards enabling us to recognize and use our own personality, in order that we may avoid the pitfalls of rejection or over-involvement in dealing with patients. The result is that we are able to become more objective in our assessment and treatment.

## Attitudes

For the Christian there are further difficulties. Failure to identify these can lead to greater tension than is necessary. The picture of the traditional atheistic psychiatrist is largely derived from Sigmund Freud and his followers. It is really just as false as the idea of the atheistic scientist of a generation ago. The latter was due to the presence of a few well-known scientists in the late nineteenth century, who were good writers for a popular readership and who spread their own radical atheism along with their discussion of current scientific findings.

Sigmund Freud was undoubtedly a genius who helped to make real progress in psychiatry. But he was first a materialist and an atheist. He expanded his psychological observations into a philosophy, and subsequently integrated his pre-conceived religious views within this philosophy. His views on religion and God have been expounded in his book *The Future of an Illusion*. In this he sees God as a projected father image in the skies. This view has been frequently discussed and answered by psychiatrists who otherwise owe much to Freud and his teaching, but who have also seen very clearly the connection between Freud's problems with religion and those which he had with his own father. Carl Gustav Jung, one of Freud's early disciples, states in his auto-biography *Memories, Dreams and Reflections* that, following a disagreement with Freud, he 'observed in Freud the eruption of unconscious religious factors'. He continues: 'Evidently he wanted my aid in erecting a barrier against these threatening unconscious contents'.

Many psychiatrists beside Freud have been interested in the immaterial part of man's nature, and have examined the beliefs and practices of their patients, including Christian and religious belief. As they seek to understand the psychological and sociological factors associated with these, they may be able to give helpful insights into the way in which certain techniques of persuasion or cultural pressures may influence a person or operate within different Christian groups. This does not mean that they can pass comment on the validity of the claims of Christianity. Here the psychiatrist is no more competent than any other specialist. Unfortunately in our contemporary deference to the expert, whatever his subject, we do not always stop to examine his credentials.

## Aims

It is because the aims of psychiatric treatment seem so close to those of the Christian Gospel that conflict arises.

We can see that medicine generally shares with the Christian Gospel the aims of helping, healing and restoring. However, where healing a limb is concerned, we can see this clearly as the province of medicine. Healing a mind, giving new purpose and strength to a person, may on the other hand seem very close to the province of the Christian Church.

Therefore the question in the minds of many Christians starting psychiatry is: 'What relevance does psychiatry have for the Christian, who believes that he has the fullest answer to man's need in the Gospel of Jesus Christ?' The question may be posed in other ways, such as: 'Will not conversion be the answer to this person's problems? or 'Should not the Christian psychiatrist seek the conversion of his patients, as only thus can they be really helped?'

Perhaps the best way to deal with these questions is to regard the psychiatrist as dealing with the mechanisms of the mind and seeking to adjust them as far as possible. The patient is one in whom the mental mechanisms have become distorted and whose mental functioning is impaired. The programme of life is going on around him, but he is picking it up with distortions. The patient's reaction to this may show itself in varying degrees, ranging from acute anxiety to madness, but his first need is for the distortions to be dealt with and eliminated. In his suffering he requires the help of a clinician, who has been trained in the special skills and techniques appropriate to mental illness.

Physical methods of treatment such as electroconvulsive therapy (ECT), phenothiazines and antidepressant drugs have, over the past thirty years, transformed the treatment of many patients. For some they have been life-saving, in others they have shortened the course of illness, and many patients suffering from chronic mental illnesses have been enabled by them to lead much more dignified and useful lives. Psychotherapy may be used alone, or in conjunction with these physical methods of treatment, to enable the patient to come to terms with the problems in his life and deal more effectively with stress and crises which occur.

In the pastoral ministry it is increasingly being recognized that many people who never reach a psychiatrist require careful and skilled counselling before, and in addition to, more direct spiritual help. The psychiatrist is increasingly being used in the training of clergy in the techniques of counselling. How much greater, then, is the need for skilled exploration and help for the person whose mind is sufficiently distressed to require referral to a psychiatrist, or admission to a psychiatric hospital. This is not to say that these people have no need of Christ; but the reason that they have rightly come to a psychiatrist is because he has the training and skills to help to restore their mental function.

It must be emphasized that all of us, as doctors, enter into a professional contract with our patient. The essence of this is that certain things are guaranteed to him. Firstly, he comes to us as doctors for our medical skill, not for our evangelism. Secondly, he trusts us to view his case with complete objectivity, unclouded by our own personal views. This professional restraint has the added advantage that the patient with a sordid life is enabled to talk about it with freedom, and the hidden resentments and hostilities of the Christian patient, which may be responsible for his present illness, are more readily explored.

Apart from these ethical considerations, that no doctor should use his professional position to impose his own views or beliefs on his patient, the psychiatrist must be additionally cautious. The success of the therapeutic relationship depends upon the psychiatrist's avoiding the temptation to offer solutions to the patient, but rather helping the patient to make his own decisions. The Christian psychiatrist (as well as the humanist psychiatrist) may explore, where relevant, the religious views or lack of them of his patient: this does not give him the right to alter them.

## Frames of reference

The Christian and the psychiatrist are both interested in man and his behaviour. But, in studying this, they may describe the same phenomena and behaviour from different frames of reference. The Christian is concerned with sin and guilt in the setting of a theistic universe. The physician specializing in psychological medicine is dealing with the experience of the sufferer in relation to his environment, and his disturbed behaviour or guilt feelings may, or may not, have underlying causes comparable to those seen by the Christian.

For the Christian, therefore, behaviour can be either 'good' or 'bad' according to how it relates to the laws of God. There are strong moral feelings expressed, and 'bad' behaviour is seen as an offence against God, a violation of what His glory demands, and is called 'sin'. So that when David sinned, he said 'Against Thee, Thee only have I sinned and done what displeases Thee.'[1] For the psychiatrist however, behaviour is often spoken of as being 'socially acceptable' or 'unacceptable', 'stable' or 'unstable'. The terms 'good' and 'bad', if used at all, are used within the context of what society permits or tolerates. As society is constantly changing in its attitudes, and at present moving away from the Biblical view of man and sin, the divergence between the Christian's frame of reference and that of the psychiatrist is increasing.

An example may be given of the way in which the Bible and society may view behaviour differently. Homosexuality is condemned in the Bible, and yet it is praised in certain great traditions. In our own culture it is tolerated now among the middle income groups, though despised by the lower income groups. We may take also a situation where behaviour may be viewed differently by the psychiatrist because of his frame of reference. A young mother is referred to a psychiatrist because of her feelings of rejection of her child. Discussion may show her to have committed adultery, desertion, child neglect, lying and theft. Theologically all this is sin; but if the psychiatrist finds that she is illegitimate, comes from a disturbed home, has had no adequate father figure or consistent affection from her mother, he may consider that he has adequate grounds for seeing this as the cause of her disturbed behaviour.   He may ask what background, instruction or model she has had from which to form acceptable behaviour, what pattern she has for becoming an adequate mother or model citizen.   Accordingly, it can be seen how her behaviour may be described as 'sinful' in the Christian context, and as 'unstable' from the point of view of the psychiatrist.

It is here that tension and anxiety arise because many Christians feel that sinful behaviour is being explained away.   In fact, only the thorough going determinist would agree that it was.   Even though the psychiatrist may describe the background and motivation of behaviour, he still holds out the possibility and hope of change.   Unstable behaviour is not inevitable, although why people should respond differently to the same backgrounds and stresses is not clear.   Certainly the psychiatrist's treatment is aimed at helping the person to change and achieve more stable behaviour.   At the same time, it is not his task to condemn or condone a person's behaviour.

## Language and terminology

A further problem contributing to communication difficulties is the use of the same words, but with different meanings.   'Guilt' is an example here.   When used by the lawyer it is something absolute and decreed, declared by jury and judge on account of proved law breaking. The feelings of the guilty party are immaterial.   Theological guilt is not exactly the same because not all sins in the Biblical sense have been declared to be crimes *by the law of the country*, for example, adultery and lying. Bigamy and slander, on the other hand, have been declared to be against the law.   In addition, there is also in theological guilt the awareness of a broken relationship and separation from God.   So the person is guilty before God, having broken His law.   He is also aware that his sin has come between him and God, and separates him from God, so that he can say with David:

'Turn away Thy face from my sins.'[2]   Only the assurance of God's mercy and forgiveness can relieve this guilt.

The psychiatrist also uses the word guilt, but he is almost exclusively concerned with *feelings of guilt*.   This is a sense of shame, failure or need of punishment, often unrelated to whether the person has done wrong at all. It may be quite unreasonable, and out of all proportion to the supposed offence, and although resisted, or confession made, it remains dominant and distressing, unrelieved by spiritual counselling or psychological treatment.   People suffering from such feelings of guilt are frequently mentally ill, and some have had to be referred to a psychiatrist by priests or ministers.   Spiritual counselling, and allowing them to dwell upon their supposed wrongs and sins, may only make them worse. Some can be dramatically and permanently relieved by modern psychiatric treatment, without losing their faith. Perhaps if William Cowper, the hymn writer, had lived today his periods of profound depression and intense feelings of guilt and rejection by God would have been relieved.   His friend John Newton, the evangelical vicar, was unable to help lift his guilty feelings.

The problem today is that, because of the very real success which psychiatrists have had in relieving some of these states of morbid guilt, there is a tendency to feel that all guilt feelings are morbid and have a pathological basis, and either require treatment or should be ignored. But most psychiatrists would admit that there are many who are referred for treatment of their 'guilt feelings', whose 'symptoms' and 'feelings' are directly related to an unsolved problem, or impaired relationship, which the patient refuses or is unable to accept or resolve.

## Responsibility

Lastly, the psychiatrist and the Christian appear to come into conflict on questions of responsibility and punishment.   Again the Bible seems clear in its statement that we are responsible for our actions before God. David said: 'I have sinned . . . so that Thou mayest be proved right in Thy charge and just in passing sentence'[3] acknowledging the freedom of man and a degree of self-determination. It is on this basis that the punishment of God is expressed and the pardon of God is offered to the man who seeks it.

Today, however, punishment is often equated in men's minds with revenge, which produces a revulsion. Accordingly there is increased pressure on the legal system to abolish the idea of retributive punishment and substitute treatment programmes for the reformation of the offender. The psychiatrist has been drawn into this debate because he found himself in conflict with the law in certain cases. The law, in its duty to protect society, was using punishment both as retribution and as a deterrent. The psychiatrist however recognized that for some offenders their law-breaking was the result of mental illness, and only treatment of their illness would prevent their committing further crime. Over the years the law has conceded the case for the brain-damaged, the insane, and the mentally subnormal. But the problem remains with those whose intelligence is normal, whose mood is stable, but whose will seems defective. They repeatedly offend and punishment seems of little help. Or again, there are those whose offence seems to arise out of unconscious or only partly conscious emotional factors, such as the middle-aged woman with no previous convictions, who shoplifts while depressed or in emotional turmoil. She may be deeply shocked and ashamed at her behaviour. Are such people not also ill and requiring treatment?

It is because of situations like these that some people wish to reject altogether the concept of responsibility and punishment in dealing with offenders. They prefer to speak of social deviation and the need for treatment. They would base their views on the belief that we cannot rightly apportion degrees of responsibility, and that punishment is not an effective way of dealing with deviants. They would say that in any case none of us is entirely responsible for our actions. There may be considerable force behind these views. It must be emphasized, however, that concepts of responsibility and punishment safeguard the freedom of the person by guaranteeing to him the dignity of freewill, and protect him from the whim of society, which after all determines deviation. Another sound reason for retaining the idea of punishment is that it is prescribed for each offence; 'treatment' may be indefinitely prolonged until the desired results is produced. It has been rightly said that the divine punishment safeguards the individual freedom of man as a responsible person – anything less makes us less human. Maybe the same is true of human punishment.

Undoubtedly there are issues here which pose considerable problems to which there seems to be no clear answer. It can be seen, however, that the Christian and psychological observations of man's behaviour are not so different nor incompatible, if it can be realized that they are couched in different language and described from different frames of reference.

The remedies for man's behaviour and condition may, on the other hand, show much less in common. This may arise from the conflict between the Christian view of man and the view of man held by certain psychiatrists. But even the Christian is only too well aware of the difficulties encountered by some in overcoming their problems of background, personality and motivation. Perhaps these issues are nowhere better illustrated than in the biography, *George Burton, A Study in Contradictions*, where a man – prominent as a Christian and evangelist in the East-end of London – is shown battling with these problems in himself.

## The Christian in psychiatry

It is a pity that some Christian doctors and medical students have tended to show suspicion and even hostility to the practice of psychiatry. In so doing, not only have they deprived the specialty of their specific contribution, but also they have left to others one of the most needy and neglected areas of patient care, especially in the field of mental subnormality. Here, I would suggest, is an area of medicine which should commend itself strongly to the Christian student and physician. For the most important skill of the psychiatrist is psychotherapy, and it has been shown repeatedly that it is the personality of the therapist which is more effective than the particular approach or school of psychotherapy. As a Christian therapist establishes a relationship with the patient, this relationship must surely be influenced by the Holy Spirit, Who is Himself dealing with the life and personality of the therapist.

Certain things, however, need to be said here. First, compassion and concern are no substitute for training and gathering experience. This process involves years of apprenticeship, supervision, and the study of associated disciplines such as psychology and neurology. It also involves higher postgraduate examinations. Second, all of us have our own personality problems, foibles and ways of dealing with stress. If we are to help others who are unable to cope with these, we must gain some insight into ourselves. Most psychiatrists gain this as they undertake psychotherapy of selected patients and discuss their progress with senior colleagues. A preparedness to examine and work through our own problems is an essential part of our training, and Christians should not expect to be exempt from this personal scrutiny and facing up to ourselves. Indeed it should be beneficial for the Christian to take stock of himself spiritually, and in every way, from time to time. He should be well prepared for this, knowing that 'the heart is the most deceitful of all things'.[4] Third, it must be emphasized again that the psychiatrist is not an evangelist or a clergyman. Although there may be considerable overlapping of roles, he should spend time working out the difference between them.

Having said this, here is a specialty in medicine which requires the physician to explore the whole life of the patient. It frequently extends his interest, involvement and healing beyond the person to his family, work and social unit. In addition, in psychiatry there is a great need to develop competence in other related disciplines, and then think across these disciplines in order to enrich the original and primary sphere. Are not such aims those which should appeal to the Christian, who has a special understanding of the family, man and society?

It is well, too, to remember that it was Christian initiative which pioneered some of the great reforms in the nineteenth century in the care of psychiatric patients. William Tuke who founded The Retreat in York, where the spiritual and moral aspects were to play as important a part as the medical in patient care, was a man who brought his Christian mind and conscience to bear upon the conditions and care of the mentally sick. It was prominent evangelicals such as Lord Shaftesbury in England and Lord Kinnaird in Scotland who championed the cause of the insane by setting up Commissioners in Lunacy. They sought to preserve the rights and dignity of mental patients as persons. It was due to men like these that British psychiatry has led the world in concern for the care of the mentally sick. To sum up, then, we may say that the difficulties in the minds of many as they start psychiatry are partly due to the novelty of the subject and partly due to apparent conflicts between the Christian and psychiatric approaches to people. The difficulties due to the novelty of the subject will be largely overcome as the student becomes more familiar with the language of the specialty, sees more patients, and understands himself better. The course in psychiatry should help him to approach people in a more mature way, and make his study and practice of medicine a deeper and more satisfying art.

Those issues which seem to point to an inherent conflict between the Christian faith and psychiatry are often due to misconceptions concerning the authority that the psychiatrist has on specific topics, or to thinking that he means the same thing when in fact he is using the same words for a different concept. Further, many people expect a complete synthesis between the Christian view of man and psychological concepts. Such a synthesis does not exist. The Christian psychiatrist must use the tools at his disposal fully realizing their inadequacies. At the same time he recognizes that here is an area where two very different 'world-view' outlooks and disciplines meet and overlap. While interested in the same people, they have only some aims in common. Mental health and spiritual life, though perhaps related, are certainly not synonymous nor necessarily dependent on each other. Consequently we still require both approaches. At the same time, we must always strive to examine and solve the problems associated with the tension points.

**References**

[1] Psalm 51:4.
[2] Psalm 51:9.
[3] Psalm 51:4.
[4] Jeremiah 17:9.

**Further Reading**

Frank J. D. *Persuasion and healing: A comparative study of psychotherapy*. London: Oxford University Press, 1961.

Hewitt D. and J. *George Burton: A study in contradictions*. London: Hodder and Stoughton, 1969.

Hooper D, Roberts J. *Disordered lives: An interpersonal account*. London: Longman Green and Co., 1967.

# 16 Specialization ✓

Philip Kennedy

THE choice of a specialty is probably the most important, and often the most difficult, professional decision that doctors are called upon to make. For a few it is readily made, but for the majority various dilemmas arise. As Christians we must at all times seek actively to participate in God's plan for us. If we do this then we are in a strong position to withstand the many tests of endurance that will beset us in our professional lives. Consequently, success and failure (and both may be repeated) will have a new significance. As training often lasts ten years or more from qualification, it must be remembered that God has work for us to do during this time, as much as at any other time in our lives.

## Choice of career

The decision as to which specialty to enter can be made at various times in one's career. It is even made, by a few, prior to undergraduate training and some decide as clinical students; but most take at least some decision, even if only in general terms, during the preregistration year for it is then that one has to decide in which of the major areas of medicine one intends to practise. It is important to decide as soon as possible partly to fulfil the requirements for specialist registration, but also to allow for the fewer hours worked under the new contract. While this has given doctors in training more free time one must accept that clinical experience will be gained more slowly. It follows that changing from one specialty to another will be more of an undertaking than in the past. Nevertheless it is equally important not to be too hasty, and firm decisions need not always be taken until after the relevant general training.

The reasons why doctors enter particular specialties are usually as varied as the applicants, but it may be helpful to consider some of them.

*Aptitude.* Personal aptitude is very important and is probably the commonest single factor dictating the choice of specialty. Some may be happy to work in non-clinical disciplines such as pathology, whereas others will prefer the close proximity to patients offered by general practice. Those possessing manual dexterity may favour a surgical specialty, while those not so endowed may choose a medical one. Those able to make rapid correct diagnoses may find themselves best suited to accident and emergency work or general practice; while those who prefer to take time in assessing a patient (I hesitate to use of them the word 'obsessional') may enter a specialty such as neurosurgery. In all this, however, we need to remember that such gifts as we possess have been given to us by God for a purpose.

*Desire to teach.* This is a common motive and a good one, but one must distinguish between a desire for self-importance in this respect and a genuine interest in imparting knowledge to others. It is, of course, a mistake to believe that this can only really be undertaken at major teaching centres. Those employed in district general hospitals can and should undertake to teach different groups of medical and paramedical workers. Opportunities of this kind have increased with the organization of Postgraduate Medical Centres, but much remains to be done. In particular, there is a great need to help the many foreign graduates now working in the Health Service who have come to this country primarily to attain postgraduate diplomas. For a variety of reasons they often hold posts in what have been referred to as 'unattractive specialties, in unattractive parts of the country' (a deplorable phrase which nevertheless conveys a meaning) and often do not get the opportunity to attend courses or ward rounds in the specialty of their choice.

In addition the ward nurses need and often would like procedures explained to them, but are sometimes too reticent to ask. Teaching should be pertinent to the needs of those being taught; the commonplace being taught before the esoteric.

*Remuneration.* The fact that it is possible (under current terms of remuneration) to earn as much, or even more, during one's professional lifetime when serving as a general practitioner than one can as a hospital specialist, means that the financial motive for entering hospital practice is no longer so attractive. The Christian doctor – following Christian ethics – should not assess an appointment solely in terms of its earning potential, nor should he choose a particular specialty because there are greater opportunities for private practice. Nor will he be interested in treating a patient simply for financial gain. He certainly will perform an operation *only* if it is clearly in the best interests of the patient.

*Research.* Research forms part of the training for nearly every specialty. But the fascination of a special form of research may draw a doctor into a particular specialty. From the Christian point of view this motive is neutral, but again the Christian doctor will wish to ensure that the patient's wellbeing overrides all considerations of scientific curiosity. If there is any doubt one should ask oneself, 'Would I be happy to have this procedure done to me or one of my close relatives in similar curcumstances?' (See Chapter 10.)

*Personal standing.* Fame used to be the goal of many

entering hospital practice. With the current and projected trends in the Health Service and in society, this is becoming more difficult to attain even for those who seek it. For the Christian the pursuit of fame should hold no attraction. It is a trap and a potential threat leading to a compromise of one's principles. This does not, of course, mean that one should not seek appointment in the most efficient hospitals or those where excellence is being achieved both in clinical treatment or scientific research. A desire to attain what one feels is the best training, or opportunity for doing the best work, is part of the production and maintenance of efficiency. The difficulty arises primarily, however, when one is seeking a permanent hospital consultant appointment, or when entering general practice. The Christian doctor may then need to make a definite choice between what most clearly follows on from what he has so far known of Divine guidance, as compared with what may seem superficially to be a more attractive course. The criterion must be God's will and the opportunity to perform the duty to the public for which he has been trained.

## Problems in training

In spite of the improvements in shorter working hours, it is still possible to become fatigued, particularly if one has heavy clinical responsibilities. Early marriage and family commitments may accentuate this problem in that they make valid demands on the limited free time available. For some, family commitments will be a reason for choosing a particular specialty; for others, the availability of married accommodation may dictate a choice of appointment. However, it is important to remember that as more senior positions are attained, the amount of time spent in the hospital is not always outside one's control. As Christians we shall wish to fulfil our responsibilities not only to our families, but to our church. These should, for example, naturally take priority over the establishment of a large private practice.

*Spiritual fitness.* During training there is a great temptation to compromise our principles in order to attain the next rung on the ladder. This fact, combined with chronic tiredness, may mean that one's spiritual life is at a low ebb. The importance of regular Bible study and prayer applies even more under these circumstances, in spite of the difficulty in securing this as a hospital resident. Sundays are frequently not off-duty days; but the Christian should not choose to do the sort of work on a Sunday which could easily be done in the week. There is, for example, no reason why regular ward or teaching rounds should take place by choice on Sundays. In any case, the patients need a day's rest even if the staff and students do not!

*Overseas work.* Specific details of training requirements for various specialties are available.[1] An interesting and important fact is that less than half the specialties listed in this Report have overseas work included in the category of 'acceptable experience'. For some doctors overseas work implies research in a North American centre or a University in one of the developing countries. Traditionally, many Christian doctors have spent several years overseas in Mission Hospital work. But with the replacement of many expatriate personnel by indigenous doctors, it is difficult for those who only have a basic general medical training (as opposed to specialist knowledge and qualifications) to find a suitable appointment, and be assimilated, other than as general practitioners, into the National Health Service when they return home. Training schemes now exist, however, to help such doctors enter general practice.

*Ethical problems.* In recent years a number of ethical dilemmas have confronted Christian doctors, for example, the 1967 Abortion Act, the availability of free contraceptives, and discussion about the use of euthana-

sia. In addition the suggestion that future appointments in obstetrics and gynaecology should be confined
only to those willing to practise a liberal abortion policy[3]
indicates one of the difficulties which may arise in
Medicine today for those who have strong ethical convictions. It is possible that similar difficulties may arise
over the problem of euthanasia, if some form of voluntary
euthanasia were to become law. (See Chapter 11.)

## The Christian view

It is right that as Christians we should desire success in
our chosen career. This does not, however, necessarily
imply that it will be in the best hospitals with rapid
promotion, security, wealth and fame. What it does,
however, imply is that we should accept God's plan for
us, and work towards it. This means that we should aim
at a thorough basic training, combined with the highest
standards of ethical behaviour towards our patients and
colleagues. We must follow what we believe to be the
will of God for us and daily demonstrate in our lives the
results of God's love for us.

### References

[1] Joint Committee on Higher Medical Training. London: Royal
College of Physicians, 1972.
[2] Report of the Committee on the working of the Abortion Act.
London: HMSO, 1974.

## 17 Christian influence in medicine: crisis or opportunity?

Alan Johnson

THE porters go on strike and patients cannot get to the X-ray department. The lift maintenance men are on strike, so it takes up to half an hour to reach operating theatres. One wonders why people work in hospitals at all. But, before the doctors point the accusing finger, they must realize that not so long ago their own junior staff worked to rule and closed some hospitals completely in order to get more pay, which no strike had done before. What is going on in medicine today? So many of the values we expected and hoped for when we started, seem to be crumbling around us. If we could see ourselves from outside, I think that we should look like a band of people hanging on to a wildly swinging pendulum and we seem powerless to stop it going too far. Unfortunately, as throughout history, when one is in the middle of a situation it is very difficult to predict how far the swing will go. It is so easy to look back once it has resolved. For example, it is now relatively easy for those who were involved to talk about the problems of living during the last War, but it was very different bringing up a young family in the middle of it, not knowing what the final outcome would be.

This uncertainty is reflected in many of the titles of

our talks and discussions – 'Crisis', 'Conflict', 'Hazard', 'Danger' – as if our only aim is to survive. Sometimes it is, but I should like to see more often words like 'Challenge' and 'Opportunity'. Every crisis is a challenge and every hazard an opportunity; and how good the Communists are at exploiting crises. Of course, Christians cannot use many of their methods; but we must analyse our situation carefully and act constructively. In the past it has sometimes taken only one man, with God's help, to stop the pendulum's swing. Even Cassius in *Julius Caesar* had to remind his colleague that 'The fault, dear Brutus, is not in our stars but in ourselves that we are underlings.' We cannot just blame 'circumstances beyond our control'. We shall always have difficult decisions to take: the whole of medicine, even on the clinical level, is a matter of trying to solve problems and as soon as one problem goes out of a bed another problem comes into the same bed!

## Recent influence

If that is what life will be like in the clinical sphere, it is going to be like that in the Christian medical sphere, too, so let us not sit back and long for a life of ease with no problems, with no challenges. Let us welcome them, accept them, and see how we can use them for Christ's sake. The whole purpose of the Christian Medical Fellowship, for example, is to relate our Christianity and our medicine – to try to stop us keeping them in two watertight compartments. We must speak and live our faith in the real world of our work. It was over twenty-five years ago that the Christian Medical Fellowship was formalized into an organization, but for some years before that graduates and Christian Unions had seen the challenge of applying their Christian faith to their profession not just in the practice of medicine but in teaching, in science and research. How are Christian doctors at present influencing the Profession? In scores of different ways; and we need to grasp again the biblical message that we are all different. We make the mistake of trying to conform to a pattern, but we have different talents, even though we are all similarly trained. Some Christian doctors are helping with sex education in their local schools; others are debating on television and radio. Some are pioneering terminal care homes or helping their local vicar's work among drug addicts. Yet others are writing to the national press about important ethical matters such as euthanasia and homosexuality. Wherever faith impinges on medicine (and that means nearly all our medical practice) we must be there, using the particular talents God has given us, because we believe that God is concerned with the whole of man and his life and his behaviour.

### Where do we start? The present climate

I suggest we must start by realizing the tremendous shift that has taken place in this country in the basis of morality over the last forty years. Those of us brought up in a Christian environment still find it very difficult to realize how pagan many people's thinking really is. Though their behaviour still conforms to the traditional pseudo-Christian pattern, they have an underlying philosophy which is rather like a hot spring bubbling under the surface: every now and then a bubble bursts the crust. In the last ten years the bubbles have been breaking through much more frequently and anti-Christian thinking has been coming out in films, magazines and television with ever-increasing force. But it has been underneath for a long time. In many ways it is easier for Christians when it does come out into the open, so that the distinction between what a Christian is and what a Christian is not, becomes very much more clear. The Christian way will become more obviously different and we shall also know what we are up against as we try to witness and speak about our faith.

It is important not to be surprised that people are anti-Christian, that we are meeting opposition, or that on the media people are saying things publicly against Christ, as if some strange thing has happened to us in this generation. Why should we be surprised? After all, we have been warned about it. Anti-Christian thought and values lead to anti-Christian actions. In the same way St. Paul emphasized that we Christians must *think* rightly if we are going to act in a right way. If, for example, you believe that a fetus is merely an appendage of the mother rather than a human being with a soul, you will act towards it very differently.

But we must realise that confusion has existed before our own era. Christianity was first preached in a society of moral chaos greater than we see in London or other big cities today. It came and challenged that society, and we are now in the position that we need no longer defend 'traditional church values'. We have been on the defensive for the last twenty-five years, but now that Christianity is no longer the 'norm' in many parts of society, we can proclaim a new way of life, a new Christian way of life, as an alternative to the atheistic and humanistic 'norm'. This, in a way, is an exciting development. We can go on to the attack instead of being defensive. However, when the early Church had a difficult problem, such as whether they should eat meat sacrificed to idols, all they had to do was to send a message to Paul and they received an epistle by return of post! It is not so easy for us and we shall have to do a lot of hard thinking, analysing and praying about these things if we are to make the right decisions and have the right influence.

There are two confusions I want to clear up before we look at these different areas. First, the *situation* may be confused. So often the situation is presented to us as a package – some good points and some bad points, in the same way as a political party has some good things which we would support and some bad things we would not support. We find it difficult to make the right distinctions when the good and bad are bracketed together: issues are not always clear-cut. For example, I may be asked, 'Is private practice Christian?' That is rather a misleading question, because private practice can be done in a Christian way, or it can be abused. Patients can be exploited in private practice and money can become the whole object of the practice. But National Health practice can be equally abused, not by making too much money from it but by not fulfilling all one's duties and treating patients as numbers. The question should be put the other way round. We should ask, 'What is the best method of payment which will benefit all so that on the one hand the patient will not be left destitute without treatment and will, at the same time, not be encouraged to be lazy? How can the doctor on the other hand be rewarded for good work and initiative, but at the same time not be tempted to exploit his patients and make a fortune at their expense?' Therefore, everything we look at, everything we meet in our practice, must be assessed in terms of the Bible to see how it measures up to Christ's teaching; which parts of it are good and which are bad, which we should support and which condemn.

Secondly, *motives* may be confused. It is so difficult to analyse our own motives, let alone those of others. When we see some employees in our hospitals with little responsibility and easy work being paid relatively more than those who work long hours and carry heavy responsibility, we are disturbed. But is this just jealousy, or is there an important principle underlying differentials between staff? Should responsibility and long training be rewarded by higher pay? These are things on which we shall have to make decisions. Again, can you really say, as a junior doctor going on strike for more pay, that you are benefiting the patient in the long run because if doctors are not paid enough there will not be any doctors to treat the future patients? Or, is that another example of mixed motives and double thinking?

## Standards for survival: progress and change

There is no doubt that for a profession such as medicine to survive, its members must show a higher standard of morality, of all kinds, than is shown in the rest of society, and its members must subject themselves to this voluntarily. Of course medicine is influenced by current social trends; but its standards must be higher. For example, if doctors stole from their patients to the same degree as many people now steal from departmental stores, the patient would not dare undress and leave his suit containing his wallet on the chair beside the couch! Most doctors *do* submit to this higher moral standard and that is why they often behave in a way indistinguishable from the Christian. A notice appeared in a magazine not so long ago advertising a 'Christian second-hand car dealer.' What was he saying by inserting the word 'Christian' here? Surely he was suggesting that, unlike many second-hand car dealers who have a reputation for dishonesty, he could be trusted. Let us hope that the Christian influence in medicine will be such that a notice reading 'Christian doctor' outside our surgeries will never be necessary! As has already been stressed, mere maintenance of the professional *status quo* should not be the Christian aim. The profession must change and change for the better but it must have a firm basis of values from which to progress or it will end by fragmenting itself and doing more harm than good.

## Distinctive Christian values

Let us now look at the basic issues in which the Christian approach is essentially different from that of the atheist or humanist.

### The nature of man

The commonly held view today is that man is merely – notice that word *merely* – a highly intelligent animal. Ideas of atheistic evolution have profoundly influenced the thinking of many people in this country. A middle-aged lady said to me during a discussion, 'Hasn't man done well in climbing up from being an ape?' What an extraordinary form of pride!

But the Christian must call attention to the fact that man has a spiritual nature and that his relationship with God is paramount. To most people, the first three chapters of Genesis are now discredited and with them the whole idea of purpose and creation. It is to be hoped that P. J. Wiseman's new book *Clues to Creation in Genesis* will help to renew the authority of the creation account. If there is no God who has created us, we have no purpose and no sense of gratitude to a Creator and it is this that leads to pride. If we do away with these chapters we discredit the idea of a Fall: so much of our sociology today is built on the erroneous principle that man is basically good and he just needs education and better living conditions to make him good. Can we really believe, as I was told recently, that all teenage pregnancies are simply due to a failure to teach the facts? Does not the *will* come into it too? There must have been a *decision*, albeit under strong emotional pressure.

Of course we must be concerned about education and living conditions. One of the troubles is that the Church at some times in the past has not been concerned with these things enough. But we must, in so doing, always remember man's basic nature. We find ourselves swinging backwards and forwards. First we have the full social gospel and we react against that. We then swing back and have no concern with social matters and preach what we call 'the true gospel'. Then we react against that a few years later, and swing back to the social gospel. We must keep the balance. Though the image of God has been marred, but not destroyed, man's nature is fallen and biased towards evil and he will not become good just by making better conditions. That does not mean, however, that we should not do everything we can to improve his conditions and to encourage social justice.

### The nature of death

The Christian must emphasize that death is not merely the end of an existence, the snuffing out of a life: there is something beyond. It is a gateway to eternity. I was most interested to hear a letter read on the radio following a discussion on euthanasia. The writer, who was not writing from a Christian point of view, said that 'the acceptance of the idea of euthanasia in our society today is due to a loss of a belief in hell'. That is because if anyone believes that when he accelerates a patient's death he is precipitating him into eternity unprepared, he will be very cautious. But if there is nothing beyond, and there is no concept of hell, then he is much happier to end that life in the same way as he is happy to end the life of a suffering dog or cat.

The Bible has much to say about hell, but I think Christians are finding it increasingly difficult to believe in and talk about it. If so, it will colour our whole attitude to death. Let us remember that it was Jesus who talked about it; the idea was not made up by some theologians a few centuries later. It was He who spoke the hard words about hell fire. Nowadays there is a reaction against the hell-fire preaching of fifty or eighty years ago, but we must keep this, too, in balance. It very much affects our attitude to our patients and to our colleagues and friends. On the other hand, the hope of eternal life means that a patient need never be left without hope. As a houseman, each time I had to certify a patient dead I used to read 1 Corinthians 15 that evening to remind myself that, for the Christian, death has been overcome and swallowed up in victory.

### The nature of responsibility

This is different for a Christian because he has a different dimension to his responsibility. He is responsible to God as well as to everybody else. Even if the relatives are not upset and the patient is unconscious, the Christian must do what is right, because he knows he is answerable to God. I am quite sure that 'The Eleventh' Commandment ('Thou shalt not be found out') is obeyed far more often today than the first, 'Thou shalt have no other gods before Me.'

The more responsibility we are given, the more it can be abused. If we do not have to 'clock in' to work, but are free to vary our working hours, that carries with it the responsibility to make up in the evening what we miss by being away during any part of the day. Many people today find it difficult to understand the New Testament principle of doing well even if there is no-one to see the result. Often the only satisfaction we can obtain from many things we do is that of knowing that we are doing God's will. God sees our motives and actions irrespective of the praise or condemnation of those around. This element in motivation is a vital ingredient in a profession such as ours. There is no such thing as rights without responsibilities. The privilege of being a doctor carries with it the duty of self-discipline. For example, we cannot carry the privilege and the responsibility of having patients' lives in our hands if we are going to drink alcohol while on duty or stay out all night before an operating list. We must finish a treatment once we have started it or, at least, ensure that someone else equally competent will do so.

There is a commonly held fallacy that it does not matter what you do off duty, it will not affect your work. This is just not true in the long run although it may seem so for a week or two. The way some members of hospital staffs spend their off duty is not always condu-cive to the spirit of responsibility they must exercise at work.

Then there is our responsibility for our colleagues. 'Am I my brother's keeper?' is the question we must continually ask ourselves. What about the conditions under which our porters and our typist/secretaries work, for example? As doctors we make a lot of the impor-tance of the conditions of work and work-satisfaction of our patients. Yet in our hospitals they put our secretaries in a typist-pool, where they never see the doctor who is dictating to them and they feel that they are working for an impersonal machine. These are the kinds of things we should be concerned about as Christians, rather than being oblivious of conditions for members of 'the team' so long as they do their job.

## The nature of love

One of the great contributions that Christianity brought to the pagan world was a new concept of love. And it needed an almost new Greek word to describe it – *agape* – charity or self-sacrificing love. Did not Jesus say 'If you love those who love you, what reward have you? Do not even tax collectors do the same? You therefore must be perfect as your Heavenly Father is perfec..' Now much present thinking in our society is built on hate. Communism is basically built on hate and envy. Even if we find ourselves working with a Communist – which we may do – on some social reform, we must never forget his driving force. Jesus said 'Blessed are the peacemakers.' It is difficult, but Heaven knows how much there is the need for peacemakers in our society and in our hospitals today. And if we look at ourselves very critically we may find ourselves taking secret pleasure at strife in other families, or in other departments, or other medical schools, because it boosts our own ego by comparison.

Martin Luther King said that love was the only force capable of turning an enemy into a friend. Do we really believe that hate can be overcome by Christian love? If so, we ought to try it out in practice. The Christian also has a new idea and a new dimension for a sexual love and relationship, and, this whole idea of self-giving love, love for no reward, is very much a *Christian* concept. Someone cynically said 'The only true charity left in the National Health Service is the Blood Transfusion Service, because it is the only thing that is done for nothing (except for a cup of tea and a biscuit!)'. For all the rest, we are rewarded pretty handsomely. Perhaps this is why the concept of self-giving and self-sacrificing love that Jesus showed so supremely, has gone out of our thinking. I recently met a Sister who had tried to arrange a blood transfusion Donor Day at her hospital and she found obstruction at every turn. No-one would help her move the benches – it was not their job. The electrician would not fix up the pumps because that was not his job. Eventually the nurses themselves had to move things around, get the room ready, and run the whole operation.

You can work in a hospital today and not exercise any love at all – either in personal relationships or to your patients – and yet appear to be a very good doctor! It was said of Lady Baden-Powell that when she spoke to you for the first time, she made you feel that she had been waiting all her life to meet you. If we could briefly convey something of that feeling to our patients in spite of the long queue outside the door, we should go some way towards showing the sort of love and concern that Jesus showed when he walked around Palestine. When He approached the blind beggar, that man was the most important person to Him at that moment.

I was given a wonderful example of this attitude by a professor of surgery in Pakistan. He would be surrounded by crowds of patients asking for his opinion as soon as he left the operating theatre to cross the courtyard. He graciously dealt with each one without showing any irritability. When I asked him how he kept so calm, he said 'Did Jesus lose His temper with the sick people who pressed around Him?'

*The nature of truth*

If Jesus said 'I am the Truth,' then Christians must take truth seriously, and it is tragic that over the years the medical profession has been identified with telling lies

175

about diagnosis and prognosis to patients. It was from the best of motives, no doubt, but the result is that patients now say 'I know he won't tell me the truth, so there's no point in asking.' Christians must work hard to get truth accepted as the norm in every walk of life. It is not an easy or a dramatic form of influence. Truth needs consistent living, consistent working, day after day. Let me give one or two examples. As the distribution of money to the various hospitals in a region depends partly on the work load of the year before, there is a temptation to return inflated patient numbers. If one hospital does this, the others instinctively react by wanting to do the same thing. It is, however, right (and pays in the long run) to put in the correct numbers and, if necessary, point out that all returns may not be so accurate. We may have to expose the unpleasant truth – let us hope that we can do it with love. If people had told the truth about the Health Service years ago we might not have several of our problems today. There is blatant dishonesty going on all around us. The amount of equipment and domestic articles that 'disappear' from our large hospitals every year is truly amazing. Often employees have the attitude that as it all belongs to a Government department it is fair game.

We must also be very definite in preventing untrue gossip and we Christians are by no means free from this temptation. I was once in a committee where a surgical registrar was being discussed and a surgeon commented 'He's a nice chap, but a poor operator.' Now I happened to have seen him operate, and had operated with him, and he was not a poor operator. So I asked if the surgeon concerned had ever seen him operate. He looked rather embarrassed and confessed he had not. That registrar's career could well have been hampered by an unfounded criticism being passed on to others.

It is difficult for Christians, because it is all too easy to speak in an arrogant way. But we have a perfect right to ask questions, 'How did you get that fact?' 'How do you know?' 'Where does that figure come from?' We must do it in that way rather than thump the table and call everybody else liars! In the same way, we have a perfect right to use all the normal democratic means to make our views known, whether it be in the Students Union or Hospital Committee.

We must be honest and truthful over our own mistakes and that's where the rub comes. Do we talk about 'a communication failure' when we mean that we completely forgot? Do we admit errors of judgment on our own part to our junior colleagues? Christians have no monopoly of this because in many places now there are meetings – on the model of American practice – when failures are discussed. Certain Christians in this country have been pioneers in this idea of actually being honest about mistakes. I once worked for a surgeon who would never have a postmortem examination, if it could be avoided, because he did not want to find out if the diagnosis had been wrong. We must be honest with *ourselves*. It is not a question of just pointing to other people's mistakes. If we are known as people who are self-critical then we have a right to be critical in other situations, provided we do it fairly and in a loving and compassionate way. Particularly we must not deceive ourselves into imagining that we are immune from common temptations, for that is the most dangerous thing of all. The Bible warns us 'Let him that thinks he stands take heed lest he fall,' but it is not the temptation in itself that is wrong – it is more often how we deal with it.

Let us relate every experience to our faith. As the hymn puts it, 'Take everything to God in prayer' – about our daily work and about our daily life. We can only do that if we realize it is not because of our own merit that we have been chosen to influence our profession, but because of God's undeserved favour.